CUMBRIA LIBRARY SERVICES

COUNTY COUNCIL

This book is due to be returned on or before the last date above. It may be renewed by personal application, post or telephone, if not in demand.

C.L.18

The ROYAL
SOCIETY of
MEDICINE

your guide to

prostate cancer

Professor Roger Kirby

MA, MD, FRCS(Urol), FEBU

Dr Claire Taylor

MB, BS, MRCS

Hodder Arnold

A MEMBER OF THE HODDER HEADLINE GROUP

Orders: Please contact Bookpoint Ltd, 130 Milton Park,
Abingdon, Oxon OX14 4SB. Telephone: (44) 01235 827720,
Fax: (44) 01235 400454. Lines are open from 9.00 to 18.00,
Monday to Saturday, with a 24-hour message answering
service. You can also order through our website
www.hoddereducation.com

British Library Cataloguing in Publication Data
A catalogue record for this title is available from the British
Library.

ISBN-10: 0340 90620 0
ISBN-13: 9 780340 906200

First published   2005
Impression number   10 9 8 7 6 5 4 3 2 1
Year   2008 2007 2006 2005

Copyright © 2005 Roger Kirby and Claire Taylor

...ed use under UK
...nay be reproduced or
...electronic or
...ng, or any information,
...nission in writing from
...opyright Licensing
...ences (for
...ned from the
...tenham Court Road,

...gsight, Manchester.
..., a division of Hodder
...1 3BH, by Cox &
Wyman Ltd, Reading, Berkshire.

Hodder Headline's policy is to use papers that are natural,
renewable and recyclable products and made from wood
grown in sustainable forests. The logging and manufacturing
processes are expected to conform to the environmental
regulations of the country of origin.

Every effort has been made to trace copyright for material used
in this book. The authors and publishers would be happy to
make arrangements with any holder of copyright whom it has
not been possible to trace successfully by the time of going to
press.

Contents

Dedication

This book is dedicated to all our patients, many of whose experiences are related here, and who have taught us so much.

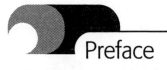

Preface

This new book, published in partnership with the Royal Society of Medicine, provides detailed, useful and up-to-date information on prostate cancer. It contains expert yet user-friendly advice, with such useful features as:

Key Terms: demystifying the jargon
Questions and Answers: answering the burning questions
Myths and Facts: debunking the misconceptions
My Experience: how it feels to suffer from, live with, or care for someone with, this condition.

Bearing the hallmark of excellence and accessibility that characterizes the work of the Royal Society of Medicine, this important guide will enable you and your family to gain some control over the way your prostate cancer is managed by being better informed.

Peter Richardson
Director of Publications
Royal Society of Medicine

Introduction

Prostate cancer now afflicts over 27,000 men every year in the UK and almost 10,000 of them will eventually die from the disease. Worldwide, prostate cancer is now the most common cancer in men and over 100,000 men die from it each year. In spite of these alarming statistics, only a minority of men are aware of the risk that prostate cancer poses to their health, and fewer still are proactive in taking steps to identify it at a stage when the disease is curable. Awareness by women about breast cancer, by comparison, is far greater and early detection and rapid, proactive treatment is now standard practice. As a result, breast cancer mortality is falling. This book aims to redress the imbalance between these two diseases in terms of public awareness and to provide in plain, straightforward language the key facts about prostate cancer, a disease that causes distress, anxiety and sorrow for so many families.

In prostate cancer especially, knowledge is power. There are now ways in which the chances of suffering from the disease can be reduced, for example, by altering the diet and adopting a healthier lifestyle. The prostate specific antigen (PSA) test, although not a perfect marker for the disease, provides an invaluable indicator of abnormal activity within the gland, but needs to be interpreted in the context of other findings, such as the size and consistency of the prostate. An abnormal reading is like a flashing dashboard light in a car – indicating that a problem is present which if fixed quickly can prevent an eventual breakdown. The exact nature of the abnormality within the gland nearly always requires a biopsy to elucidate. This can usually be done as an outpatient procedure, with only minor discomfort providing that generous local anaesthesia is used. The interpretation of the biopsy results, particularly the so-called Gleason score, which is the best indicator we have of the likely future behaviour of any cancer present, is subtle and depends on the experience of the pathologist (the doctor who looks at the biopsy specimen down the microscope), and a second opinion on this may sometimes be warranted. CT (computerized tomography) and MRI (Magnetic Resonance Imaging) scans, as well as a bone scan, may also be necessary to ascertain whether or not the disease has spread beyond the confines of the gland.

Often the most difficult part of the prostate cancer 'journey' is the decision about which treatment option to select. In the past this diagnosis used to be accompanied by the initiation of hormone therapy that effectively meant the end of an active sex life and eventual recurrence of the disease. Now a bewildering array of treatment options exist, including potency preserving surgery (with or without laparoscopic and robotic assistance), brachytherapy, conformal radiotherapy and high intensity focused ultrasound (HIFU). In addition, it is now recognized that some cancers are sufficiently small and grow so slowly that no treatment at all is needed, and instead 'active surveillance' can be employed. In more advanced cases hormone treatment is required, but now the option exists to take a daily tablet as opposed to monthly or three-monthly injections. Moreover the tablets have a less severe impact on sexual function.

The decision about which treatment choice is right for which individual is not always an easy one, and needs to be taken with as much impartial advice and clearly understandable information as possible. Men who embark on prostate cancer treatment empowered by knowledge and who are supported by their families suffer less stress during therapy, are more positive about their outcome and often seem to fare better as their illness progresses. We hope that this book will help to make the prostate cancer journey a little easier to travel for all those concerned.

CHAPTER

1

What causes prostate cancer?

The prostate gland is a chestnut sized (20 cc) organ found only in men. It sits just below the bladder and surrounds the urethra or tube that drains the bladder through the penis (see Figure 1.1). Its job is to produce PSA, a substance that liquefies the jelly-like substance that sperm are stored in so they can swim towards and fertilize the egg.

Prostate cancer, like other cancers in the body, develops as a result of a series of genetic faults. Each of these tiny copying errors in the genes that control cell growth, progressively builds on the last one until, eventually, the cell's behaviour is altered. Normally, cells divide only when the body needs them to, and the process is under strict control. When this genetic control breaks down and the cells begin dividing in an unregulated manner, a mass of excess cells forms, known as a **tumour**. A tumour can be classified as **benign** (non-cancerous), or **malignant** (cancerous). It becomes cancerous when the uncontrolled, rapidly dividing cells acquire the ability to invade the surrounding healthy tissue. Because of this ability

tumour
A collection of cells that increases in number outside the body's normal control. Tumours may be cancerous or non-cancerous (benign).

benign tumour
A growth that, although increasing in size outside the body's control, can't invade the surrounding structures or spread elsewhere inside the body.

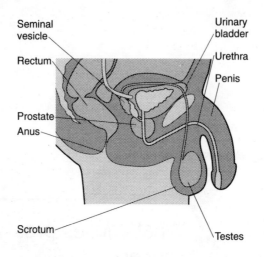

Seminal vesicle
Urinary bladder
Rectum
Urethra
Penis
Prostate
Anus
Scrotum
Testes

Figure 1.1 The anatomical location of the prostate gland.

malignant tumour

The medical term for what is commonly called cancer. In malignant tumours the uncontrolled cancer cells are invading normal surrounding healthy tissue and have the potential of forming metastases. A malignant tumour has the ability to kill a person.

metastases

This is when cancer cells travel through the bloodstream or the lymphatic system to other parts of the body and settle there. The word 'secondaries' is often used instead of metastasis.

of prostate cancer to invade surrounding areas, it can spread by direct invasion to sites around the prostate gland and, at this point, the prostate cancer will be termed 'locally advanced'. As the cancer becomes larger it also becomes more dangerous as it can spread through the bloodstream or lymphatics (tiny channels that drain fluid from the tissues) to other areas of the body to form secondary cancers or '**metastases**'. At this stage the disease may become life-threatening, gradually taking over the body, unless treated.

myth
Cancer is always a death sentence.

fact
Wrong. Although some men will die of their prostate cancer, with better detection and treatment increasing numbers of men can be cured. Prostate cancer is a slow growing cancer which is curable in some men, while in others the disease can be controlled for prolonged periods of time. Furthermore, the many men who are diagnosed with prostate cancer will in fact die as a result of another incidental condition, such as heart disease, rather than their prostate cancer.

When prostate cancer spreads and forms metastases or secondaries, small clusters of cancer cells break off from the main tumour in the prostate and enter the bloodstream and **lymphatic system** (the latter is a network of tiny vessels that drains fluid from all the organs in the body). In this way, the prostate cancer cells are transported to other parts of the body and, like seeds in fertile soil, settle and start to grow. In the case of prostate cancer the two most common sites in which metastases form are the bones, especially of the spine and pelvis, and the lymph nodes. In contrast, benign tumours such as **benign prostatic hyperplasia (BPH)** can still cause problems from a squashing effect as they increase in size but they will not spread (metastasize) to distant sites, and consequently are seldom life-threatening.

lymphatic system
This system of small vessels drains fluid (lymph) from the body's organs, filters it and returns it back to the bloodstream.

benign prostatic hyperplasia (BPH)
A benign or non-cancerous condition that causes the prostate gland to swell up. BPH, like prostate cancer, can cause difficulty in passing urine.

Q **What are the first signs of prostate cancer?**

A This is difficult to answer as there is a spectrum of first signs and each man will be different. In some men the prostate cancer is an incidental finding, that is, before the patient has any ill effects, due to a raised prostate specific antigen (PSA) blood test taken by a doctor. In some men they may experience increasing difficulties in passing their urine or find they are passing urine very frequently. Finally, some men will have no real changes to how they pass urine but will feel generally run down with weight loss and pains in their bones.

PSA (prostate specific antigen to give it its full name) is a protein produced by all prostate glands whether healthy or not. If the prostate has a cancer in it or is inflamed because of infection, the amount of PSA detected in the blood rises. PSA readings, in the form of a blood test, are used by doctors to help diagnose prostate cancer and monitor its response to treatment. Chapter 5 further explains PSA, its uses and some of the problems with it as a diagnostic tool.

Stages of prostate cancer

If prostate cancer is suspected in a man, tiny samples or **'biopsies'** of tissue from the prostate gland will usually be taken and sent to a **pathologist** for analysis. The method by which the prostate biopsy is taken is called a transrectal ultrasound (TRUS) biopsy and will be fully explained in Chapter 4. The pathologist will examine the biopsy under a microscope and, if a cancer is seen, will endeavour to answer two questions: how much of the sample has cancer in it and how aggressive is the cancer likely to be? Both of these pieces of information are very useful to the doctor and patient in planning treatment. As well as information from the prostate biopsy, the PSA reading and various scans show how far, if at all, the cancer has spread outside the prostate gland and will help the team to guide the best type of treatment to select.

biopsy
The removal of a small sample of any body tissue for analysis. Biopsies are usually taken to see if there is cancer present or not.

pathologist
A doctor who specializes in looking at the structure of tissues microscopically. Pathologists play an important role in diagnosing and guiding the treatment of cancer.

Prostatic intraepithelial neoplasia (PIN)

The earliest stage in uncontrolled prostate cell growth is not actually classed as a malignancy or cancer, but as a 'pre-malignancy' or 'pre-cancer', known as prostatic intraepithelial neoplasia (PIN for short). PIN can be found on its own, or in combination with prostate cancer when examining prostate tissue under the microscope. PIN is characterized by a 'heaping up' of cells within the prostate, but there is no invasion of healthy tissue at this stage. With time, however, these dividing cells may develop the ability to invade normal prostate tissue, hence, becoming a cancer in the process. These early signs of invasion give the pathologist looking at the sample of prostate tissue a hint that an actual cancer has developed from the pre-malignant PIN. At this stage, the level of the glycoprotein substance known as PSA in the blood often also begins to rise above the normal value of 4 ng/ml (**nanograms per millilitre**) – another important clue that prostate cancer is developing.

nanograms per millilitre (ng/ml)
This is a measure of concentration that is used in PSA tests. The PSA figure is in fact the amount of PSA in nanograms seen in 1 millilitre of blood.

As prostate cancer develops, it eventually forms a distinct lump or 'nodule' within the gland that can then grow and spread locally to other structures that lie close to the prostate gland, such as the **seminal vesicles** and the capsule that surrounds the prostate. Please refer to Figure 1.2 on the anatomy of the prostate to find out more about where these structures are located.

seminal vesicles
A pair of storage vessels for sperm, found just behind the prostate gland and often one of the first areas that prostate cancer spreads to.

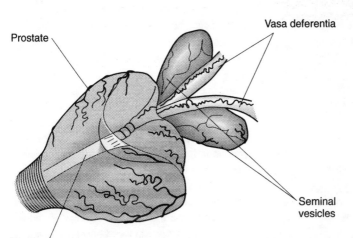

Vasa deferentia

Prostate

Seminal vesicles

Urethra

‖ **Figure 1.2** The anatomy of the prostate gland showing various seminal vesicles.

differentiation
When healthy prostate is seen under the microscope a pathologist will easily recognize it as coming from the prostate gland. This is 'well differentiated' tissue. As cancer takes over the prostate, cancer cells can lose some of their characteristic prostate features. These cells are now 'poorly differentiated' and unrecognizable from any other cancer.

Gleason grading system
Developed by Dr Gleason, this is an international system of grading how abnormal prostate cancer cells look under the microscope. The grades run from 1 to 5, and the higher the grade the more aggressive a cancer is likely to be.

Gleason score
Prostate cancer is not uniform in Gleason grade. Therefore it is common to note the grades of two areas in the biopsy sample, for example, $2 + 2 = 4$. Again, the higher the score the more aggressive the prostate cancer is likely to be.

As prostate cancer grows, the cells it is composed of change or mutate, becoming increasingly abnormal and therefore less identifiable as prostate tissue when the pathologist looks at them down a microscope. This process is known as '**differentiation**' and was described in the 1960s by a histopathologist called Dr Gleason. He devised the now universally accepted **Gleason grading system**, according to the shape, size and structure of the cells in the prostate sample, that is still used today. Because prostate cancers are not uniform throughout the gland, the Gleason method assesses the two most prominent groups of cancer cells within the sample separately, and then the two separate grades are added together to give a '**Gleason score**'. The two most prominent groups of cancer cells are selected and graded by inspection of all the prostate samples available under a microscope.

The Gleason grade of the prostate cancer cells varies from 1 to 5; the higher the number, the more aggressive the behaviour of the cancer. Grades 1 and 2 prostate cancer are sometimes termed 'well differentiated' as the cells are still easily identified as stemming from the glandular tissue of the prostate. Conversely, Gleason grade 5 is 'poorly differentiated' as the sheets of highly malignant cells are difficult to identify as coming from the prostate if seen in isolation. As mentioned above, the two most prominent patterns are usually assessed, and the two grades added together to give what is known as the Gleason score. In the overall Gleason score, where the grades from the two test samples are added together, the score will vary between $2 + 2 = 4$ and $5 + 5 = 10$. In summary, the higher the score (from 4 to 10), the more aggressive and potentially dangerous the cancer is likely to be. The Gleason score will be one of the main factors that will be taken into account by the medical team, the patient and the family when deciding which type of treatment is most likely to cure, or at least delay, the spread of the prostate cancer.

As has been pointed out already, prostate cancer cells can develop the ability to invade surrounding healthy tissue and also spread locally and beyond to bones. The extent to which this has occurred is known as the clinical stage of the cancer. How far and to where the cancer has spread is another key question that will influence treatment. Once prostate cancer cells have developed the ability to invade healthy tissue, they initially infiltrate locally within the prostate gland itself. The cancer slowly grows larger, buried within the prostate, until it reaches the surrounding capsule. Small cancers cannot usually be felt during a physical examination. The best way to detect these small cancers is by means of multiple biopsies, usually under ultrasound vision via the back passage (rectum). Larger cancers can usually be felt during an examination via the rectum, a test known as a digital rectal examination or DRE, which is described in detail in Chapter 4. The ease with which a prostate cancer can be felt through the rectum depends not only on the cancer's size but also on its position within the prostate.

---

myth
Cancer is a single disease.

fact
Cancer is a condition that can affect any organ in the human body but in each of these places it will look and behave differently. Some cancers grow faster than others while some will be more aggressive, spreading to other areas of the body early. This diversity is further underlined by the various treatments that have been developed. For some, surgery is the best option while for others drug treatment (chemotherapy) or radiation works better.

Q **In the first stages of prostate cancer, is there any discomfort to warn you?**

A We are afraid not – this is part of the tragedy with prostate cancer. When the cancer is still small and confined to the prostate gland it rarely causes any trouble to the man, who remains unaware of the cancer.

For example, a cancer developing towards the back of a man's prostate will form a lump or nodule which can be felt during an examination much sooner than one growing deeper inside the gland. Increasingly localized prostate cancers may not be detected on DRE but are diagnosed purely on the basis of an abnormal PSA test.

Metastatic (secondary) prostate cancer

At first, the prostate cancer spreads locally to tissues around the prostate, most notably the capsule of the gland and the seminal vesicles, which lie behind the prostate and contribute secretions to the ejaculate. Eventually, however, it may spread to more distant sites, such as the lymph nodes, lungs and bones (see Figure 1.3). The mechanisms by which the life-threatening ability to spread ('metastasize') is acquired by the cancer cells are currently the subject of intense scrutiny by scientists. Research is currently being undertaken into various aspects of this process. This ongoing work includes the study of how the prostate cancer metastasis establishes its own blood supply (a process known as 'angiogenesis') at the distant site and what makes it settle at certain preferred sites, notably within the bones. It is hoped that if we understand some of these processes better, we can then develop treatments to prevent the spread of prostate cancer. At present, many men with prostate cancer only visit their doctor when their prostate cancer has already spread (that is, when it is 'metastatic') and although it is still controllable in the short term, by that stage regrettably it is seldom completely curable.

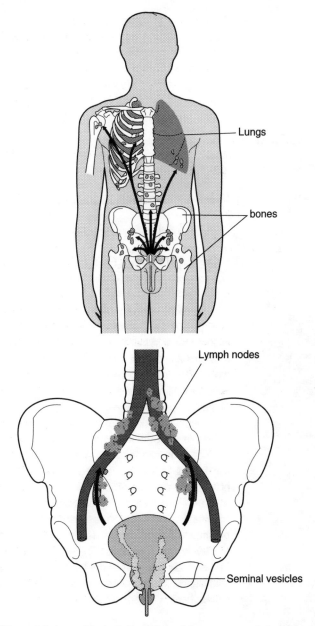

Lungs

bones

Lymph nodes

Seminal vesicles

Figure 1.3 Areas of the body to which prostate cancer can metastasize (spread) – the lymph nodes, lungs and bones.

CHAPTER

2

Why do some men get prostate cancer?

Overall, each and every man runs something like a 10 per cent risk of developing prostate cancer at some point in his life. The lifetime risk of dying of a prostate cancer is thankfully rather lower at around 3 per cent. However, these are average figures for all men. Each individual man's chance of getting prostate cancer will depend on his own personal **risk factors**, some of which are avoidable (**modifiable**) and some of which are not (**non-modifiable**). A good example of risk factors is seen in heart disease; a family history is a non-modifiable risk factor, whereas smoking is an entirely avoidable, and hence modifiable, one. Of course there are also **protective factors**, which lower the likelihood of developing a specific disease. In the case of heart disease this would include lowering cholesterol, keeping slim and physically fit and eating healthy foods (such as those low in saturated fat).

Risk factors are characteristics or actions that influence the chances of that person developing a specific disease. It should be remembered that even if a man has more than one of the risk factors listed below it does not guarantee that he will eventually develop prostate cancer. It just means that his chances are greater compared to a man without those specific risk factors present.

Of course, it is always a good idea to lead a healthy lifestyle, eat a well-balanced diet and keep physically fit to prevent a host of medical conditions.

Risk factors associated with prostate cancer

The following factors may play a part in increasing a man's chance of getting prostate cancer:

✧ Belonging to an older age group (50 years +)
✧ Having one or more close family members with prostate cancer
✧ Belonging to certain ethnicities (for example, Afro-Caribbean)
✧ Eating a diet high in fat
✧ Having low sunlight exposure.

Age

The most important risk factor for developing prostate cancer is increasing age. Prostate cancer is rarely seen in men aged under 40 years, yet is common in men over 60 years. Studies have shown that the average age of death from prostate cancer within the UK is around 70 years. Considering the overall average age at death is now 77 in men, this means that seven years of expected life are lost – precious retirement years that most men have anticipated all their working lives.

protective factors
Things that may protect a man from getting prostate cancer, for example taking selenium and vitamin E supplements.

myth
Having a risk factor means you will definitely develop prostate cancer.

fact
This is not the case. If you have one of the risk factors that we talk about in this chapter it means that you have a higher chance of developing prostate cancer but this is not a guarantee you will develop it. Remember that if it is a modifiable risk factor you should make an attempt to eliminate it.

myth
All old men have prostate cancer.

fact
Prostate cancer is a disease of older men but with the vast majority of men with problems passing urine, it is because of the non-cancerous swelling of prostate called benign prostatic hyperplasia (BPH).

first degree relative

This is basically your parents or your brothers and sisters, providing they have the same parents. In the case of prostate cancer, a disease seen in men only, we are only interested in fathers and brothers.

second degree relative

This is anyone once removed from the first degree relatives, for example, grandparents, aunts and uncles. Again, in prostate cancer we are only interested in the male second degree relatives.

genes

These are the smaller building blocks of chromosomes. There are millions in every chromosome. Each gene can be responsible for forming a specific characteristic, chemical or protein within the body.

chromosome

Each cell has 23 paired rod-like chromosomes which are responsible for the transmission of hereditary characteristics.

Family history

Prostate cancer can run in certain families, just like breast cancer. A man who has a brother or father (medically known as **first degree relatives**) or an uncle or grandfather (**second degree relative**) who was diagnosed with prostate cancer before their sixtieth birthday has a two to three times greater risk than a man with no affected relatives. Furthermore, if there are several first degree relatives who have been diagnosed with prostate cancer the risk may be higher although this has not yet been proven in studies. For this reason specialists try to identify these families so that male members can be carefully monitored, usually in the form of a regular PSA test, to diagnose any cancer early on. It has been observed that men in these 'prostate cancer prone families' tend to develop relatively dangerous and aggressive prostate cancers at a fairly young age.

It is estimated that around one in ten cases of prostate cancer may be family based and the result of a problem in the **genes** handed from parents, particularly fathers, to sons. Each and every cell in our bodies holds a set of 23 paired **chromosomes** packed with genes that control the cells' development and functions. We all have different chromosomes, half from our mother and half from our father, making each and every one of us unique. The idea of an inherited prostate cancer has sparked a lot of interest, and many resources and much effort have been channelled to look into this phenomenon more deeply. Results so far have pointed to problems in two different genes. A mutation, or fault, has been located on a specific gene (short arm of chromosome 1q, to be precise) as well as a prostate cancer 'susceptibility' gene which is located on the male sex chromosome. Other suspect genes are currently being studied for potential prostate cancer inducing faults.

Unfortunately, at present we are unable to alter someone's genes to reduce the risk of them developing prostate cancer. However, we can be more vigilant in detecting the cancer early in affected men and their family members. In practice this means regular screening for a rise in the PSA and early recourse to biopsy.

my experience

I am an accountant who happens to be an identical twin. When I was 54 I learnt that my twin brother had been diagnosed as suffering from prostate cancer and had undergone surgery for this in the United States of America. I immediately consulted a urologist who organized a PSA, which indicated that I was borderline at 3.6 ng/ml, and a biopsy which revealed one core positive for adenocarcinoma. My staging scans were negative and after lengthy discussions with the medical team about my various options I opted for a radical prostatectomy. This was carried out successfully, and examination of the prostate by the pathologist confirmed complete excision with no evidence of disease. Post-operatively the PSA decreased to less than 0.1 ng/ml and remains undetectable during follow-up.

Race

Men of Afro-Caribbean race have a higher risk of prostate cancer, which tends to afflict them at a younger age than Caucasian men. Afro-Caribbean men also seem to develop the more aggressive, higher Gleason score prostate cancer. Conversely, men of Far Eastern extraction seem relatively less likely to be affected by the disease.

Testosterone

The male sex **hormone**, **testosterone**, is essential to normal prostate growth and development as well as the changes of puberty.

hormones

Chemical messengers that travel through the bloodstream. Hormones allow different bits of the body to communicate with each other. Usually hormones influence processes at a different site from where they are produced.

testosterone
The hormone responsible for many male characteristics. It has a role in stimulating growth of prostate tissue, so some drugs used in prostate cancer work by disrupting its production or blocking its effect.

Following puberty, testosterone levels vary widely from man to man with no effect on their masculinity. It has been observed that men castrated before they enter puberty, so-called 'eunuchs', never develop prostate cancer. However, there is no clear link between either high or low testosterone levels in fully mature men and the development of prostate cancer, although research in this area continues.

Reducing the risks

Diet

The first of the avoidable risk factors is a high level of saturated animal fat in the diet. A man worried about his risk of prostate cancer (or indeed heart disease) is well advised to limit his intake of eggs, milk, cheese, butter and red meat. It is thought that foods high in saturated animal fats increase the levels of free radicals in the body which have the ability to damage the genetic material in the body, thereby increasing the chances of prostate cancer.

There is some evidence that certain dietary supplements may offer some protection against prostate cancer. Preliminary studies suggest that both vitamin E and selenium are also antioxidants that reduce free radicals and hence protect against cancer. It has also been reported that lycopenes, which are found in tomato skins, are protective against prostate cancer, although more work is required to confirm this. Obesity is also strongly associated with prostate cancer, so staying slim and fit is also a useful way to decrease the risk of the disease.

If men wish to take dietary supplements, the advised dose of vitamin E is now 100 international units per day, selenium 200 micrograms per day and lycopenes 15 milligrams per day. (*If you want to take a vitamin or mineral supplement, it's a good idea to check with your GP (general practitioner) first; some ingredients can interfere with medicines that you might be taking, or affect an existing medical condition.*) Furthermore, a diet rich in fruits and vegetables, especially tomatoes and berries, may be helpful in preventing the disease.

Specific medicines which may help prevent prostate cancer

In a very large trial the drug Proscar™ (also known as finasteride), which acts by preventing the conversion of testosterone to its more active form within the prostate, appeared to reduce the risk of prostate cancer by a quarter. Unfortunately, those cancers that did develop in the men on Proscar™ seemed to be more aggressive in nature than those in the placebo (dummy drug) group. More work is being done in this area as a similar but newer medicine Avodart™ (dutasteride) is also undergoing trials for what has been termed preventative activity. Very recently it has been reported that cholesterol-lowering drugs known as statins may reduce prostate cancer risk. More work, however, is required to confirm this.

UV light

Geographically, prostate cancer tends to become more common as you move away from the equator; Norway and Sweden have the highest death rates from the disease worldwide. This fact points us to two further possible modifiable risk factors – low vitamin D and low exposure to sunlight, which itself helps the body to produce vitamin D. Regular holidays in the sun therefore seem like a good idea!

myth
Prostate cancer is a sexually transmitted disease.

fact
This is not true. There is no link between any sexually transmitted disease and prostate cancer. Furthermore, prostate cancer cannot be 'caught' from other people or toilet seats.

Environmental factors

Men who work with cadmium and in the nuclear power industry have been found to have a higher incidence of prostate cancer when compared to the general population. However, the exact cause of this observation is unknown, although it may be due to accumulation of radioactive heavy metals within the prostate. Other pollutants in the environment, such as pesticides, may also be partly responsible for the recent rise in numbers of men suffering from prostate cancer. Another possible culprit is bisphenol A, a chemical widely used in the food industry to make polycarbonate drinks bottles and the resins used to line tin cans. New research suggests that small amounts of this chemical entering the diet could have a negative effect on the developing foetus in pregnant women. Because the chemical mimics the impact of the female sex hormone oestrogen, its impact on the prostate would only show up years later in the form of a greater susceptibility to benign or malignant disease.

CHAPTER

3

The symptoms of prostate cancer

Increasingly nowadays people are taking greater interest in their health. This is reflected in the fact that more and more people are tying to eat a more healthy diet and take regular exercise to prevent disease. For example, a generation ago vitamin and mineral supplements or products aimed at lowering cholesterol were not widely used, but now they are part of a burgeoning 'health market'. Furthermore, people are learning more about their bodies and what can go wrong. Increased media interest in conditions such as breast cancer in women and, to a lesser extent, prostate cancer in men, has heightened awareness in the general population and more and more information is available on the worldwide web. This has benefits in that people are living longer than ever before and also consulting their doctors earlier if they feel something is wrong. Unfortunately, however, men tend to be less well educated about their health than women, and are much more reluctant to go to the doctor, unless a pressing reason presents itself, or their partner insists!

symptoms

These are the problems that men with prostate cancer notice that prompt them to go to see a doctor. Symptoms are often regarded as a change from the normal. With prostate problems, the commonest symptom people suffer from is increasing difficulty in passing urine and the need to visit the toilet more often, especially at night. Discomfort develops as a result of incomplete bladder emptying.

signs

These are the changes in the body, caused by a disease, which a doctor will pick up as he or she examines the patient. Some are easy to see or feel as they are on the surface of the body, for example, a swelling in the groin. Some involve an internal organ that may need special scans or tests to pick up.

As a result of increasing media attention and publicity, however, an increasing number of men are consulting their doctors with minimal or no urinary **symptoms** at all. This can happen either because they are worried about prostate cancer, or a health check has turned up an abnormality. Yet there are still many individuals who do not present for medical help until they are suffering from widespread metastatic (secondary) prostate cancer.

In this chapter we will discuss some of the commonly seen symptoms and **signs** of prostate cancer. Please remember though, that no two people are the same, and men with prostate cancer are unlikely to have a 'full house' of the symptoms described below. Men who are suffering from some of these symptoms should also bear in mind that commonly occurring non-cancerous conditions in the prostate and bladder can cause similar effects. If you are worried that any of the descriptions given may apply to you please go to your doctor and ask for a check-up.

Men with prostate cancer but no symptoms

Men in this group will not be aware that there is anything wrong with their prostate, as they have not noticed any changes in their health or their body. Generally men who see a doctor in the absence of symptoms fall into one of three camps. First, there are those who have consulted their doctor as they are worried about developing prostate cancer. Not uncommonly, these men have a relative or close friend who has prostate cancer or they have become worried after reading or hearing about prostate cancer. Second, there are those who have gone to the doctor about an unrelated problem or who have attended a health insurance or work medical and the suspicion of prostate cancer has been raised. In these men it is usually the case that the doctor did not think the prostate was normal on examination or that there was an abnormality in the PSA blood test. PSA blood testing is discussed in greater depth in Chapter 5, as interpreting the results can be tricky.

Q **Can I get checked for prostate cancer even though I have no symptoms?**

A If you have any worries about prostate cancer, please make an appointment to see your doctor who will check you out. He or she will ask questions about any symptoms and why you have your concerns. They will examine you, including doing a DRE and perform a PSA test, provided that you understand the implications of the test.

Finally, there is a third group of men that deserves a mention in this section. These are men who have surgical treatment for non-cancerous prostate enlargement and an unexpected cancer is found. Benign (non-cancerous) prostate enlargement is far more common than prostate cancer itself and, again, increasingly affects men as they get older. Indeed studies have shown that 50 per cent of 60-year-olds and 90 per cent of 80-year-olds suffer from this condition.

Treatment, initially, is often by tablets but a proportion of men have an operation known as a transurethral resection of the prostate (TURP) that cores out the inner most part of the prostate. The net result of this operation is that the passageway through which the bladder empties is opened up again. As in all operations, the

myth
You have to have symptoms to have prostate cancer.

fact
When a prostate cancer is developing within the gland, initially it is very small and will not distort the gland in any way. Because of this it will not cause any problems to the man and hence you can have prostate cancer and not feel anything is amiss.

prostate tissue that is removed is sent to a histologist to confirm that there is no cancer. In less than 10 per cent of such men some small areas of cancer are found. When this happens the rest of the prostate gland is usually assessed by an ultrasound performed via the back passage (rectum) and biopsy as well as a PSA measurement. The details of both of these tests are explained more fully in Chapters 4 and 5.

Symptoms from an enlarging prostate gland

When cancer develops inside a prostate gland it enlarges which, in turn, causes the gland to swell, or distorts its shape. The prostate gland is found just below the bladder and has the urethra – the tube that runs from the bladder down the penis through which a man urinates – in fact passing straight through the middle (see Figure 1.1). So the prostate completely surrounds the channel for drainage of the urine held in the bladder. Therefore, it is not difficult to imagine that if the prostate is swollen and distorted it can squeeze on the urethra and thereby hamper the process of passing urine. When this happens most men notice a characteristic set of symptoms, which doctors call 'obstructive symptoms', which are listed opposite. The most common of these is a weakening stream when urinating, but the stream may also become intermittent or even reduce to a series of dribbles, especially at the end of the stream. Another common obstructive symptom is that of difficulty initiating urination despite the bladder being full. Finally, sometimes men with prostate problems don't feel they have emptied the bladder fully despite their best efforts. When this gets very severe complete retention of urine may occur, requiring urgent treatment by catheterization (the passage of a small tube into the bladder to allow the urine to drain). The following are all common symptoms:

✧ **Weak stream** is a reduction of the force and strength of the stream as a man passes urine. It tends to be a gradual decline in the force over time.

✧ **Hesitancy** is the term used to describe the scenario when a man has to wait seconds or even minutes at the toilet to start urinating despite him feeling he wants to go. Often men strain to pass urine at this point.

✧ **Intermittency/post micturition dribbling** is when the stream of urine stops and starts and finishes with dribbles and drips rather than cleanly.

✧ **Incomplete emptying** is the feeling that urine remains in the bladder despite the fact the man has stopped passing urine.

The second group of symptoms is related to irritation of the bladder and results from the straining it is doing to push urine through the narrow urethra. Unsurprisingly, doctors tend to call this group of symptoms 'irritative symptoms'. The most common of these is the need to get up multiple times at night to empty the bladder ('**nocturia**'). Men with prostate cancer may also find they have to go to the toilet with more **frequency** during the day. Sometimes men suffer from so-called '**urgency**'. When this happens they have a very strong desire to empty their bladder that may send them running to the toilet. What can be particularly frustrating for these men is that when they go to the toilet the amount of urine passed seems very small to cause such a strong desire to empty the bladder. These symptoms result in what is known as an overactive bladder, which can be very debilitating.

It should be remembered that all the symptoms described above may be seen in both

> **nocturia**
> The need to get up and pass urine multiple times during the night despite cutting down on the amount of fluid consumed during the evening.

> **frequency**
> The need to empty the bladder at regular intervals during the day. The amount of urine may be large or small.

> **urgency**
> A sudden overwhelming desire to empty the bladder. People often think they are on the verge of wetting themselves and will run to the toilet. Other men describe urgency as suddenly feeling like they have more urine in their bladder than they could possibly hold.

non-cancerous and cancerous conditions of the prostate and bladder. If a man is experiencing any of them, he should be encouraged to go to his GP for a check-up. If deemed appropriate the GP will then refer him on for a specialist opinion.

my experience

When I was aged 62 I found I needed to get up several times during the night to go to the toilet, but when I got there I experienced a reduced urinary stream. I refused to consult my doctor as I was far too busy at the time and also didn't want to trouble the practice. Eventually my wife prevailed upon me to seek help. Although my GP expected the diagnosis to be benign prostatic enlargement, when he examined my prostate via my back passage, he could feel a sizeable hard lump. He checked a PSA value which came back at 62 ng/ml and arranged an urgent outpatient opinion from an urologist. Biopsy of the gland confirmed that I had prostate cancer and a CT scan suggested that it had spread to my lymph nodes. I was also found to have secondary tumours in my lung. Surprisingly the bone scan was clear. I was immediately started on hormone therapy and my symptoms have improved and my PSA has fallen to normal levels. I am now in remission.

Symptoms from the local spread of prostate cancer

Although to begin with a developing prostate cancer grows within the prostate gland, it can begin to invade the capsule and spread to the tissues surrounding the gland over time. Each man's prostate cancer differs in its characteristics and, as a consequence, there are no fixed rules as to when, and even if, the prostate cancer will spread. The location of the cancer within the prostate gland will play a part in whether it spreads locally. If the cancer is near the surface of the prostate gland it does not have to grow that much to distort and then spread through the surrounding capsule of the gland. Those cancers that lie buried deep within the prostate gland generally have to grow larger before they reach the surface capsule of the gland. The fact that prostate cancers are often multiple suggests that the entire gland is unstable and therefore more susceptible to cancerous change. When the prostate is removed, although there is usually one dominant lump, there are very often smaller subsidiary tumours present.

Local spread is the term used to describe the situation when the cancer has grown and directly invaded through the surrounding capsule of the prostate and is infiltrating out into the structures and tissues surrounding it in the pelvis. Prostate cancer that has spread locally is essentially all part of one large mass that has escaped the confines of the prostate gland. The symptoms that a man will suffer from with local spread are a reflection of what structures the prostate cancer is invading. This can include the bladder, the back passage or rectum and the nerves that control erections or skin sensation in the groin or the area behind the scrotum.

If the cancer has spread upwards into the base of the bladder, the patient may suffer from the same irritative symptoms described in the last section. These include nocturia, frequency of urinating and urgency of urination. Furthermore, if the cancer is invading the muscle wall of the bladder the patient may see blood staining of his urine, which can range from a pale pink colour to bright red with clots. Finally, in some men the flow of urine from the kidneys to the bladder can be disrupted by a blockage of one or both of the ureters (the paired tubes that connect the kidneys to the bladder). When this happens the kidney becomes engorged and swollen with trapped urine and, if left for a long time, the kidney will not work normally even after it has been unblocked. If both ureters are blocked, no urine can be passed and kidney failure will rapidly occur.

> **local spread**
> When the prostate cancer grows and breaches the capsule of the prostate gland and spreads into the surrounding tissues.

> **myth**
> If you have problems passing water you have prostate cancer.

> **fact**
> This is not true. Non-cancerous benign prostate hyperplasia (BPH) infection in the prostate (prostatitis) and problems with the muscle of the bladder can all give the same symptoms as prostate cancer.

If the cancer has infiltrated the nerves coursing through the pelvis, the resulting irritation can cause a range of symptoms. For example, a nerve responsible for skin sensation in the groin or the perineum (the bridge of skin between the scrotum and anus) will signal its irritation by pain or, less commonly, numbness in those areas. Sometimes the nerves that stimulate and co-ordinate erections are affected and a man will notice either a reduction in strength or complete loss of erections. Cancer invading the seminal vesicles, paired structures around the back of the prostate gland that store sperm (see Figure 1.2), can result in blood being seen in the ejaculate ('**haemospermia**'), a rather alarming symptom that is more usually associated with a stone, or a recent biopsy of the prostate, or stones, within.

haemospermia
This is where blood is mixed in with the sperm and is seen once it has been ejaculated at the time of orgasm. It can be a sign of prostate cancer but also of stones or an infection in the urinary system.

Symptoms resulting from metastatic disease

Unfortunately, approximately one-third of men with the disease still do not consult a doctor until after the prostate cancer has spread throughout the body. When a cancer has spread either via the bloodstream or lymph system, small new deposits of cancer can start growing almost anywhere in the body. The lymph system is a network of small vessels that can transport white blood cells that fight infection and are also used to drain excess fluid from the tissues back to the heart. As both blood vessels and lymph glands contain fluids that circulate around the body, the cancer can, conceivably, settle anywhere. In reality there seems to be certain tissues that prostate cancer has a preference to settle in, namely the bones, the liver and the lungs and more rarely the brain (see Figure 1.3).

Secondary cancer deposits in the bones, or 'bony metastases' to give them their medical

myth
All prostate cancers develop at the same pace and metastasize at the same time

fact
All men are different and it is difficult to predict which men will have small prostate cancers that grow very slowly and never leave the prostate gland and those unlucky men with aggressive prostate cancers growing and spreading rapidly.

term, often cause pain. The most common place for a bony metastasis to develop is in the pelvic bones and spine, but they can sometimes be found in the ribs or the long bones in the arms and legs. As well as causing pain, a bony metastasis can weaken the structure of the bone causing it to fracture (a **pathological fracture**), often with very little precipitating force. Occasionally when there are many cancer deposits in the spine, the spinal cord running down the centre can be pressed upon resulting in a condition known as '**spinal cord compression**'. Spinal cord compression may cause weakness in the legs and loss of control of the bladder and bowel sphincters that prevent leakage of urine and faeces. Eventually complete paralysis of the lower limbs may develop.

Secondary prostate cancer deposits in the liver tend to cause discomfort and pain in the upper part of the abdomen, particularly on the right-hand side. If there is a large volume of cancer in the liver then it cannot function properly and the patient may turn a yellow colour and become '**jaundiced**', as one of the waste products the liver usually breaks down is deposited in the skin.

In addition, as with all patients with advanced cancer, there is a range of non-specific symptoms caused by the cancer generally upsetting the body's overall balance. These include tiredness or malaise and lack of energy as well as loss of appetite and loss of weight.

pathological fractures
A break through an area of bone weakened by a prostate cancer metastasis.

spinal cord compression
This is when a bony metastasis in the spine compresses the cord containing the major nerves that run through it. It will result in loss of sensation and power in the legs and sometimes loss of bladder and bowel control.

jaundice
The yellow discoloration of the skin that occurs when the liver cannot do its job of clearing toxins from the body. Metastases from prostate cancer can cause a failure of the liver as they replace the normal tissue.

CHAPTER

4

The diagnosis of prostate cancer

Seeing a doctor

For most men the first medical practitioner they will approach with their concerns is their GP, although they may also trawl the internet or call NHS Direct (see Further help). The GP will want to know the reason for the visit and will ask about the presence of the symptoms as described in Chapter 3. If the man is requesting a PSA blood test to screen for prostate cancer in the absence of any symptoms, the GP will often enquire about the reasons for this. Although a GP cannot refuse to take a PSA blood test on a man who is requesting one, he or she has a duty to ensure that the man realizes the consequences of a positive result and understands that a marginally raised PSA is not always due to cancer in the prostate. PSA testing and screening is a matter of some controversy both within medical and public health circles. We have therefore devoted Chapter 5 to the contentious issue of the PSA test together with its advantages and disadvantages.

Regardless of the reason for a man's attendance, as well as asking about any problems with urination, the GP will usually want to examine him physically. First the GP will ask the man to lie on an examination couch so that he or she can feel his abdomen. The reason for this is because if there are problems emptying the bladder and urine is being left behind, the bladder can become so distended that it is felt protruding out of the pelvis. Normally, a doctor can't feel the bladder when pressing from the outside as it lies behind the bones of the pelvis, but when the bladder is very full it can be palpated through the soft muscle of the lower part of the abdomen. The next thing the GP will do is examine the **external genitalia** of the patient. The genitailia consist of the penis, testicles and scrotum. Before starting the examination the doctor will explain what he or she wants to do and will ask the patient's permission. He or she will look at the penis and the scrotal skin and then gently feel the testicles within the scrotum to make sure there are no abnormal lumps or swellings.

The final and most important part of the examination is a **digital rectal examination (DRE)**.

Digital rectal examination

This is probably one of the things about prostate assessment that men feel most concerned about. A digital rectal examination (DRE) is undeniably a little uncomfortable, however it is over quickly and can give a doctor valuable information about the prostate. Again, the doctor will explain what he or she is going to do and will try to reassure and relax the man they are about to examine. The doctor will ask the man to adopt a specific position for the test. Most doctors ask the man to

external genitalia
The medical term for the sexual organs, comprising the penis, scrotum and testicles in a man.

digital rectal examination (DRE)
This allows the doctor to assess the size and texture of a man's prostate gland. It involves placing a gloved and lubricated finger in the man's back passage to feel the gland.

fact
It is undeniable that many men feel uncomfortable and embarrassed when a doctor performs a rectal examination. However, to the doctor a rectal examination is just another part of a physical examination and he or she will not see it as something unpleasant, dirty or sexual. Try to relax and it will be over before you know it.

roll over on to his side and to bring his knees up to the so-called 'foetal' position (this is because it is the position that we were all in when we were in the womb). While in this position the doctor will gently insert a gloved finger, which they will have lubricated with some KY jelly, into the man's rectum (see Figure 4.1). To do this the finger is pushed through the anal sphincter and therefore the more relaxed the man is the easier it is to do this. Often breathing in long, deep breaths, closing the eyes and trying to relax can help make this less uncomfortable.

When the doctor is performing a DRE he or she is able to feel the posterior (or rear facing) part of the prostate gland through the rectal wall. The normal prostate is roughly the size of a chestnut. The doctor will determine if the gland feels symmetrical and of a soft consistency.

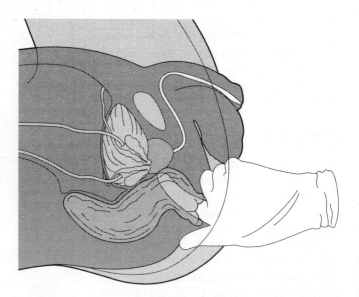

Figure 4.1 Digital rectal examination of the prostate.

Hard, craggy consistency, nodules, lumps or asymmetry can all point to the presence of cancer in the prostate gland. Occasionally another abnormality, such as a polyp or an ulcer in the rectum, is detected, and a **referral** to a rectal specialist will be arranged.

The whole thing is over in less than a minute or two and when it comes down to it most men agree that a trip to the dentist is much more uncomfortable!

referral
A process where one doctor asks a fellow doctor, usually of a different speciality, to review a patient and offer help in their diagnosis or treatment.

Seeing a specialist

Urologists are specialist doctors that look after disorders of the kidneys and bladder in both sexes and the prostate and external genitalia in men. **Urologists** are mainly hospital-based doctors that perform surgery as well as looking after people in the **outpatients'** department. The GP will usually refer a man to a urologist if they find a high PSA (usually greater then 4 ng/ml) or feel there is an abnormality of the prostate on examination. Less commonly the referral will be to an **oncologist** (a doctor who deals with all types of cancer).

It is vital that the man trusts and relates to his specialist team completely because if a cancer is diagnosed he will want to feel confident in the advice and treatment that he is receiving. The doctor–patient relationship is a two-way thing; as well as the specialist giving advice about treatment, the patient should be comfortable enough to ask questions or discuss treatment options that they may have learnt about through other sources. The specialist should give clear explanations of any tests and their findings as well as going through the various treatment options for prostate cancer and their advantages and disadvantages for that individual's problems. He or she may suggest a meeting with a urology nurse specialist. If, for whatever reason, a man

urologist
A doctor that specializes in disorders affecting the kidneys, bladder and, in men, the prostate.

outpatients
This is when you travel to a hospital to consult with a specialist at a booked time. It does not require you to stay in hospital.

oncologist
A doctor that specializes in the medical treatment of cancer.

with prostate cancer does not feel confident in the specialist team he has been referred to, he should go back to his GP to discuss the problem or call one of the helplines mentioned at the end of this book. His GP will review the case and often recommend a second opinion from an alternative urologist or oncologist. Some men with prostate cancer choose to consult a specific doctor privately because of their reputation or as a result of a personal recommendation. If this is the case, and it is to be done through private healthcare insurance, please remember to check the policy and call your insurer before booking the appointment, as some policies require a GP referral first.

Diagnostic tests

The specialist may go back over some of the ground already covered by the GP, as this information is often better first hand. They will ask the patient questions about how well they are emptying their bladder as well as some background questions on their general health. The examination will be repeated as well. The PSA blood test is often repeated, as it is useful to know if this is rising rapidly or remains relatively steady. Urologists also often ask for a more informative special form of PSA test called the 'free to total ratio'. Please refer to Chapter 5 for more information on PSA testing and its variations.

A number of other tests may be recommended which may include:

✧ A physical examination to check the patient's general state of health (including a DRE). Blood pressure (BP), pulse, height, abdominal girth and weight may also be checked.

✧ A urination questionnaire to be completed by the patient himself which will give information on any urinary symptoms and will provide the specialist with an International Prostate Symptom Score (**IPSS**). However, remember these symptoms can be due to prostate cancer or BPH.

IPSS

The international prostate symptom score is a standardized questionnaire that specialists may ask a man to fill out so they can assess how bad the urine symptoms are.

✧ Blood tests to assess blood and kidney function. By taking around two tablespoonfuls of blood, the test can determine whether there is adequate haemoglobin (red blood cells, lack of which causes **anaemia**) and normal blood urea and creatinine, as these can both deteriorate with prostate cancer if the kidneys are obstructed. Other results such as blood sugar and cholesterol level may be used as indicators of general health. This is especially important if either surgery or radiotherapy is being considered as a possible treatment alternative.

anaemia

The medical term for having a low blood haemoglobin level. Anaemia can cause tiredness and shortness of breath on exertion.

✧ A urine test to check for bacteria, as there may be a urinary tract infection (UTI), and/or blood, as this can develop if the prostate cancer is causing obstruction or has spread into the urethra or bladder. Very recently a urine test which is collected immediately after a vigorous massage of the prostate has been described. The massage releases prostate cells which can be collected in the urine and analysed for their genetic characteristics. Early results suggest that a recently discovered gene known as UPM3 may be helpful in distinguishing those men who do harbour prostate cancer from those with benign enlargement of the prostate.

transrectal ultrasound scan (TRUS)

An ultrasound method that allows the prostate to be seen. It involves inserting a lubricated probe into the back passage to visualize the prostate gland. It is used to guide biopsies or brachytherapy treatment.

Prostate biopsies and transrectal ultrasound scanning (TRUS)

If cancer is suspected by the specialist, he or she will usually recommend biopsies of the prostate; first to confirm that there is cancer present and, second, so that the prostate samples removed can be graded according to the Gleason score. As mentioned in Chapter 1, grading of the cancer provides valuable information about how aggressive the cancer is and helps to guide the patient and specialist about the optimum treatment.

The taking of prostate biopsies involves two constituent parts: a **transrectal ultrasound scan** (**TRUS**) and the taking of the biopsies themselves. Having been given some antibiotics (either as a tablet or injection) the patient will be instructed to adopt the same curled up lateral 'foetal' position that is used during a DRE.

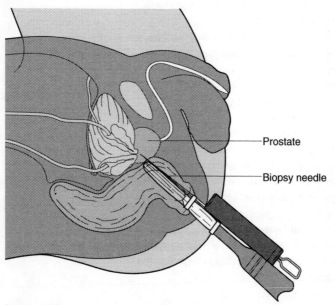

Prostate

Biopsy needle

Figure 4.2 Transrectal biopsy of the prostate.

A lubricated and sheathed, ultrasound probe, not much larger than a finger, will gently be introduced into the rectum (see Figure 4.2). The high frequency sound waves emitted from the probe bounce off the surrounding structures back to the probe. A computer can use these echoes to produce an image of the prostate on the screen. Again, irregularity in the shape or consistency of the prostate or deficits in the capsule are noted and the size of the gland calculated.

Prior to the taking of the prostate biopsies a local anaesthetic is usually injected around the prostate capsule. Don't be afraid to ask your doctor about this, as the anaesthetic considerably reduces the discomfort associated with the procedure. A biopsy is uncomfortable but not very painful, although the sharp individual needle pricks can usually be felt as the special biopsy 'gun' is fired. The biopsy needle is inserted through a special port in the ultrasound probe and then advanced into the prostate under the TRUS guidance. Between 6 and 12 cores of prostate tissue are removed as tiny samples from representative areas of the gland. Furthermore, if there is a particularly suspicious area seen on ultrasound, this will be specifically targeted. The prostate biopsies will then be carefully labelled and sent to the pathologist for expert examination and interpretation.

Oral antibiotics are continued for several days after the test. Sometimes blood can be seen in the urine, semen or bowel motions for up to four weeks following the biopsies. This is to be expected, but any concerns should be communicated to the doctor. Finally, there is a small risk of developing a urinary tract infection after the procedure, which is why antibiotics are given to all patients in an effort to reduce this complication. If the urine becomes cloudy or

myth

Transrectal ultrasound and prostate biopsies hurt.

fact

Again, this is not a pleasant experience, but the information from the prostate biopsy will be vital to your specialist to guide the best treatments. It is uncomfortable but should not cause pain. Injections of local anaesthetic or lubricating gels with added local anaesthetic are used to try to remove as much discomfort as possible.

smelly, if there is burning and frequency of voiding or if the patient feels unwell with a high temperature, a doctor should be informed and he or she will probably prescribe more antibiotics. Very occassionally the patient will develop shaking attacks (rigors) and might need to be admitted to the hospital to receive antibiotics intravenously via a drip directly into a vein. If you have any worries after a prostate biopsy, do not hesitate to call your doctor or the hospital where the procedure was undertaken. The results of the biopsy – either positive or negative for cancer – should be available within a few days or weeks of the investigation. Again, don't be worried about asking when the results are expected to be available. Obviously this is critical information for the patient and his family.

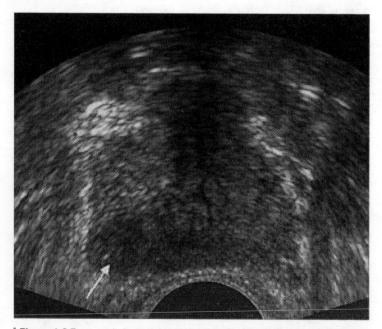

Figure 4.3 Transrectal ultrasound scan showing a prostate tumour (arrowed).

my experience

I am a 54-year-old accountant who underwent a transrectal prostate biopsy as an outpatient to investigate the cause of a slightly elevated (5.4 ng/ml) PSA. I was prescribed antibiotics for 24 hours before and 48 hours after the biopsy. The procedure was uneventful and relatively painless because of the use of generous quantities of local anaesthetic. Two days after the biopsy I began to feel unwell and developed a high temperature. I called my GP who arranged for me to be admitted to hospital. Intravenous antibiotics were given and blood cultures taken which revealed an infection in the bloodstream due to bacteria known as E. coli. However, I made a rapid recovery and the biopsies showed benign changes in the prostate with no evidence of cancer.

myth

Transrectal biopsies of the prostate can cause the cancer to spread through the body.

fact

Untrue, there is no evidence that the small biopsy needles used to obtain specimens from the prostate gland cause the disease to spread. In fact it is the nature of the cancer itself that determines the tendency for a given cancer to metastasize and form secondary tumours. The greater the Gleason score and the higher the PSA value at diagnosis the greater the chances are that spread has occured or will occur.

Staging tests

Cancers, as well as being **graded** for their aggressiveness are also 'staged'. **Staging** aims to identify how far the prostate cancer has spread. This is a second vital bit of information required for planning the treatment of prostate cancer. Some treatments are better suited to cancer confined within the prostate gland and some are able to treat prostate cancer in the surrounding tissues or once it has spread to distant sites (metastasized).

The most common notation for this assessment is the tumour-nodes-metastasis system (TNM system for short). The TNM system can be applied to any cancer and is internationally agreed. In the case of prostate cancer the tumour stage runs from T1, a small focus of cancer deep in the gland, to T4, cancer that has spread from the gland into the pelvis (see Figure 4.4). If there is evidence that the prostate cancer has spread to the lymph nodes in the pelvis or beyond it is termed N1, if there is no lymph node spread then N0 is used. The same principle applies to metastasis, M1 if they are present M0 if not.

grading

This looks at the prostate cancer cells themselves to assess how aggressive the prostate cancer is likely to be.

staging

This looks at how far a prostate cancer may have spread outside the prostate gland.

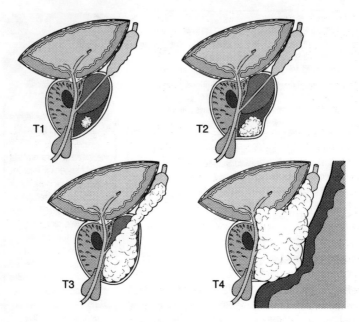

T1

T2

T3

T4

▌**Figure 4.4** Clinical staging of prostate cancer.

Bone scan

bone scan
Radioactive markers are used to show up whether there is any prostate cancer deposits in the bone and if so where they are.

A **bone scan** checks to see if the prostate cancer has spread to the bones, the most common place for prostate cancer secondaries to metastasize to. A bone scan will not always be done as men who are diagnosed early with a very small prostate cancer and relatively low PSA result are very unlikely to have bony spread. Several hours before the scan the man with prostate cancer will receive an injection. The injection is of small weakly radioactive particles (radioisotopes) that are then allowed to circulate in the bloodstream. Bone metastases have a rich blood supply relative to the surrounding bone and therefore when the scan is done with a machine that picks up the radioisotopes any bony metastases show up as 'hot spots'. Don't be concerned about the use of radiation here – the dose is so low that the risk to health is negligible.

Computerized tomography scan (CT scan)

A **CT (computerized tomography) scan** uses an X-ray machine that looks like a very large polo mint and can take pictures from 360 degrees. The person lies on a table that passes through the hole in the middle of the scanner as the pictures are taken. A computer then takes all the X-ray pictures and amalgamates them so that the doctors can look at pictures representing 'slices' through a person. As these are X-rays and not real pictures the detail of the prostate gland is not perfect. CT scans are used to look for enlarged lymph nodes in the pelvis which may have prostate cancer in them or, rarely, can be used to guide a biopsy of a suspicious lump in the pelvis. Some specialists who are planning to perform surgery (radical prostatectomy) like to send their patient for a CT scan before the surgery to be sure that the disease has not spread outside the gland. A CT scan is also used to plan the dosage of radiation to be used in radiotherapy of the prostate.

> **CT (computerized tomography) scan**
> A method of using sequential X-rays to build up a three-dimensional picture of the body.

Magnetic resonance imaging (MRI)

This is similar to a CT scan in the sense that it takes images from 360 degrees and a computer reconstructs them into slice type pictures. The main difference is that instead of X-rays the effects of a strong magnet on the body are used. The scanner is more like a tunnel and some find it rather claustrophobic. Again, **MRI scans** can be

> **MRI scan**
> This stands for magnetic resonance imaging. This builds a three-dimensional reconstruction of the body. Unlike a CT scan, MRI detects very small movements in the bodies cells when they are exposed to a magnet for a short period of time.

used to look for lymph node spread and some of the new scanners can give greater detail of the prostate and the immediately surrounding tissues than a CT scan. However, biopsies can't be performed in a MRI scanner and anyone with a metal implant, such as a coronary stent or a pacemaker can't be exposed to the strong magnetic field it uses. A recent innovation known as MRI spectroscopy produces images that show most precisely the location of the cancer. This information, taken in conjunction with the clinical stage, the PSA value and the biopsy result, provides a better estimation of the extent and the location of the tumour and helps the patient and doctor together to arrive at correct treatment decision.

my experience

I am 73 years old and have had a pacemaker fitted as well as a total hip replacement on my right side. A little while ago I noticed I was having trouble passing water with a very poor urinary stream. I also noticed that I occasionally had blood in my urine. I went to my doctor who carried out a PSA and then sent me off for a biospy. The biopsy confirmed prostate cancer but luckily a bone scan proved negative. Because of my pacemaker I could not have an MRI but a CT scan confirmed a locally advanced tumour without evidence of spread to the lymph nodes. After I discussed various treatments with the doctors involved, as well as my family, I decided to use a seven-week course of conformal radiotherapy preceded by three months of hormone therapy to pre-shrink the tumour and improve my response to radiation. So far I seem to be responding well to treatment and the tumour seems to be shrinking and my PSA has fallen.

CHAPTER

5

Prostate specific antigen

Even though doctors have routinely used prostate specific antigen, or **PSA**, for over 15 years to test for and monitor prostate cancer, PSA testing remains a controversial topic. The main reason behind the controversy is that all healthy men have some PSA in the bloodstream and raised levels of PSA are not exclusively caused by prostate cancer. Therefore, best medical practice is always to confirm a suspected diagnosis of prostate cancer by looking at the suspected cancer cells under the microscope in a sample of prostate tissue that has been obtained in a biopsy. That said, some men have their prostate cancer diagnosed solely because of a raised PSA test and this is achieved before they know anything is amiss. These men have a greater chance of being cured by any treatment, as the cancer is usually small and still contained within the prostate gland.

This chapter highlights some of the advantages and disadvantages of PSA testing. When it comes down to it, there are no right or wrong answers as to when or why men should request a PSA test.

PSA (prostate specific antigen)
PSA is a protein produced by all prostate glands whether healthy or not. If the prostate has a cancer in it or is inflamed because of infection, the amount of PSA detected in the blood rises. To help diagnose prostate cancer and monitor its response to treatment, doctors use PSA readings in the form of a blood test.

We hope that having assimilated the information and discussed it with their families, men will be able to form their own views and if they want to take a PSA test they can go to see their GP knowing that they understand the arguments both in favour and against PSA testing.

What is PSA?

ejaculation
The emission of about a teaspoonful of sperm with a nourishing fluid at the point of orgasm.

PSA is a glycoprotein found in abundance in every man's ejaculate. It is made in the prostate gland and added to the sperm to make the semen liquid after **ejaculation** and thus promote fertilization. In a healthy prostate gland the cells making up its structure fit closely together and therefore very little PSA leaks out of the prostate gland and into the bloodstream. However, there is always a small amount of leakage and therefore men with an entirely normal prostate will have a low level, usually described as <4.0 ng/ml (nanograms per millilitre), of PSA in the bloodstream.

Q If my PSA is above normal will they automatically send me for a biopsy?

A If your PSA is raised the first thing that will happen is that you will have an appointment with the specialist to discuss the implications and what happens next. The majority of men with raised PSA go on to have biopsies to definitively diagnose or rule out prostate cancer. In a few men the PSA may be monitored for a period of time to look at the trend. However, if this is the case, the specialist will explain the plan and reasons fully to you.

The basis of the PSA test

In a healthy prostate gland the PSA glycoprotein is manufactured and mixed in with the sperm just before it is ejaculated at orgasm. If it has been a while between orgasms, PSA makes it way through special little drainage tubes (ducts) into the urethra. Once in the urethra it will be washed out the next time the man passes urine.

If there is any disease affecting the prostate gland, be it infection, inflammation, trauma or cancer, the watertight arrangement of the cells lining the gland becomes disrupted and PSA can leak out into the bloodstream. Of all the processes named above, the most damaging to the prostate by far is cancer. As a prostate cancer grows, it invades the surrounding cells and destroys them, causing progressive damage and, in turn, allowing increasing amounts of PSA to leak into the bloodstream.

PSA in the bloodstream is detected by a simple blood test, taken from a vein in the arm. Less than 5 ml of blood (one teaspoon) is needed to perform the test in an automated analyser machine. The machines available to measure PSA usually take a few hours to give a result. Obviously, if repeated PSA measurements are required it is best to have them at the same place so the same machine is used, but this is not essential.

Causes of a raised PSA test

It is generally accepted that the upper limit normal for a PSA blood test is 4 ng/ml, although some experts now argue that 2.5 ng/ml is a better cut-off value. (A cut-off value implies that men with a PSA value above the cut-point are at risk of prostate cancer while those with a PSA below the cut-point are in the clear.) Studies of healthy men, with no prostate problems, have shown that there is a tendency for the PSA level to fluctuate a little from day to day. Although the PSA is not constant it should not display a continued upward trend or increase above 'normal levels' and that finding serves as a trigger for further investigation. Therefore, any man with a PSA level of 4 ng/ml or above on testing is said to have a raised PSA and by definition some sort of prostate problem (either benign or malignant). As mentioned above, there are several different factors that can cause a raised PSA and it should be emphasized again that cancer is only one of them.

First, there is a condition called benign prostatic hyperplasia (BPH), which affects men far more frequently than prostate cancer, especially as

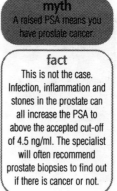

myth
A raised PSA means you have prostate cancer.

fact
This is not the case. Infection, inflammation and stones in the prostate can all increase the PSA to above the accepted cut-off of 4.5 ng/ml. The specialist will often recommend prostate biopsies to find out if there is cancer or not.

they get older (see Chapter 1). As the name suggests, this is a non-cancerous swelling of the prostate gland that can cause similar problems with urination. As the prostate enlarges it can cause a modest, progressive rise in the PSA leakage into the bloodstream. Indeed, in the absence of cancer the PSA value can give a useful estimate of how enlarged the prostate is as a result of BPH.

A second prostate problem that can temporarily cause a raised PSA is inflammation of the prostate, either because of infection in the prostate gland or in urine, or prostatic stones, which are small, calcified deposits in the gland. This tends to cause a transient increase in PSA as once the cause of the inflammation is treated the PSA will usually settle.

Third, any trauma to the gland will temporarily disrupt the architecture of the prostate and cause temporary leaks of PSA. The most common cause of trauma is, in fact, a doctor undertaking prostate biopsies or passing a **catheter** up the penis into the bladder. Furthermore, any prolonged pressure on the **perineum**, the area behind the scrotum and in front of the back passge, can cause minor trauma to the prostate. Studies on the Tour de France cyclists have shown that they have a significantly raised PSA after sitting on their narrow bicycle saddles and pedalling furiously all day!

There is no evidence that stress, diet or alcohol can influence the PSA level. Nor does a gentle DRE alter the PSA value, but recent ejaculation may result in a minor rise.

It is therefore apparent that PSA tests are only prostate specific, rather than prostate cancer specific. A raised PSA means there is some form of prostate trouble, but does not always mean that it is cancer. This is why a PSA blood test alone is not enough and the doctor's questions as

catheter

A narrow tube inserted into the penis and up to the bladder to drain urine away. The tube is connected to a bag that will collect the urine as it drains. Catheters can be used temporarily after operations or in the longer term if required.

perineum

The area of skin situated behind the scrotum and in front of the anus.

well as a careful examination of the prostate by rectal examination are also a must to put the PSA value in context.

my experience

A couple of years ago, aged 51, I was told I had an elevated PSA of 7.4 ng/ml after a routine check. I was immediately referred for transrectal biopsies of the prostate which proved negative. I was reassured but it was suggested that I went for a further PSA test in six months' time. When this was done, alarmingly, a further rise of PSA to 9.8 ng/ml was detected. I was sent off for further more extensive biopsies which revealed two cores from the relatively inaccessible anterior part of the prostate which showed evidence of cancer. Staging scans luckily showed no sign of disease outside the prostate. I decided to opt for a radical prostatectomy which was performed successfully and pathological examination of the specimen revealed a sizeable tumour in the anterior part of the prostate with no extension beyond the surgical margins. Since then, the PSA test during follow-up has remained undetectable at less than 0.1 ng/ml and I'm feeling positive about the future.

Medical reasons for doing a PSA test

From the general public's perspective it is widely believed that a PSA test is only used to diagnose prostate cancer, mostly due to the not always helpful media coverage. However, PSA levels can have several uses in the diagnosis of prostate conditions, in selecting and monitoring treatment and in predicting the progression of prostate disease. They can also be helpful in deciding between treatment options for men with a benignly enlarged prostate.

The one-off PSA level, as an indicator of cancer in the prostate gland is the most heavily promoted use but it does have its drawbacks (see page 48). As well as helping to diagnose prostate cancer, the PSA level can also be used to monitor the

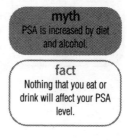

myth
PSA is increased by diet and alcohol.

fact
Nothing that you eat or drink will affect your PSA level.

effectiveness of its treatment. No matter what treatment a patient receives for his cancer, the PSA level should drop and then plateau at a much lower value. Every patient is different and there is no specific number that is aimed for in all cases. The PSA is normally taken regularly, usually every three months initially and then every six months after a year or so. When using PSA as a monitoring test, it is the overall trend that is important; if the PSA progressively increases with time, the doctor will want to make sure there has been no recurrence of the prostate cancer, which would then require reassessing the treatment plan, and perhaps changing medication or employing other treatment alternatives such as radiotherapy.

In conclusion, measurement PSA levels have been shown to be helpful in guiding diagnosis, treatment and follow-up of both cancerous and non-cancerous abnormalities of the prostate. In the BPH there are two different types of drug that can be used to improve the urinary problems. Studies have shown that the size of the prostate on DRE and the PSA level can guide doctors as to which of these two treatments is likely to work best. Avodart™ (dutasteride) and Proscar™ (finasteride) are most effective in men without cancer who have a prostate larger than 30 ccs in size and whose PSA is greater than 1.4 ng/ml. Alpha blockers such as Flowmax™ (tamsulosin) or Xatral XL™ (alfuzosin) seem to work to improve symptoms and flow regardless of the size of the prostate or the PSA.

myth
You cannot request to have a PSA test

fact
Every man has the right to request a PSA test from his GP. A GP can't refuse you, but they will ask you your reasons and discuss the implications of having the test and the result being abnormal.

How is the PSA test being made more predictive of prostate cancer?

This is an area of much scrutiny by scientists, urologists and oncologists. They are constantly looking into ways to make the PSA test a more accurate way to diagnose prostate cancer. So far, several ideas have been put forward, many of which have been researched at great length, but unfortunately the foolproof test for prostate cancer still eludes us. Below are some of the more common ways that PSA readings are evaluated to make them more accurate in diagnosing prostate cancer.

◇ **PSA density**

This attempts to get around the problem mentioned above that large but non-cancerous glands could leak as much PSA into the bloodstream as a small cancer in an otherwise normal sized gland. It is calculated by dividing the blood PSA reading by the volume of the gland as shown on a transrectal ultrasound scan. The higher the PSA density the more likely there is cancer in the prostate.

◇ **PSA kinetics**

As the name suggests, PSA kinetics is the rate of increase in PSA year on year. Again, this tries to separate the non-cancerous from cancerous conditions in the prostate. If there is cancer in the prostate the PSA tends to rise more rapidly than with the other prostate problems. Recent data suggests that men with a PSA rise of more than 2 ng/ml a year before diagnosis are more likely to harbour clinically aggressive prostate cancer.

◇ **Age related cut-offs**

These were developed because older men tend to have bigger prostates than younger men and having the same normal PSA range for a 40-year-old and an 80-year-old seemed illogical. Table 1 (on page 46) shows the accepted age-related PSA readings, which get higher as a man ages.

Table 1

Age	PSA cut-off
40–49 years	2.5 ng/ml
50–59 years	3.5 ng/ml
60–69 years	4.5 ng/ml
Over 70 years	6.5 ng/ml

✧ **Free to total PSA ratios**

These came about following an observation that scientists made when studying the PSA molecule. In the bloodstream, PSA is bound to a specific type of protein that stops it causing damage to other constituents. For reasons that are not clear, in men with prostate cancer the amount of unbound or 'free' PSA is reduced. As a consequence, a reduction in the percentage of 'free' PSA can be an early warning sign for prostate cancer. The cut-off point is usually taken at 18 per cent.

Deciding whether to have a PSA test

When it comes down to it, PSA testing, like so many other things in life, is not perfect but it does have some real advantages. Any man, as well as those close to him, needs to decide whether they are happy to risk the problems with PSA testing to allow as early a diagnosis of prostate cancer as they can achieve. When a man is considering whether to ask for a PSA test, the information below may help him to come to a decision. There are no absolute right and wrong answers and every person will have their own opinion and preferences. Patients will usually find it very helpful to discuss this with their GP, urologist or nurse specialist who may also ask some questions about symptoms and perform a DRE to allow a more informed decision. A great deal of helpful information on this subject is also on the web. Try, for example, www.prostate-research.org.uk

The main disadvantages of PSA tests stem from the fact that it is not a prostate cancer specific marker. This chapter repeatedly mentions 'cut-off' levels which are based on large studies of men both with and without cancer. If a man is one side of this magic number he has prostate cancer but if he is on the other he hasn't. This means that some men will have a small prostate cancer but a PSA on the non-cancerous side of the cut-off, and conversely some men will go for prostate biopsies to confirm prostate cancer when there is in fact none there.

The advantages are easy to spot – PSA testing can save lives. If there is a cancer a man has a much greater chance of being cured if it is small and confined to the prostate gland. Furthermore, these men often have yet to notice any problems with their urinating or any ill effects from the cancer.

The advantages and disadvantages are listed below but we would urge men to discuss the decision to have a PSA test with their loved ones as well as their doctor, urologist or specialist nurse.

Pros of a PSA test

◇ Allows early detection of a potentially curable prostate cancer
◇ Negative tests are reassuring
◇ Repeated PSA tests can be used to monitor the effectiveness of prostate cancer treatments or surveillance in higher risk individuals

✧ If a patient is subsequently found to have
BPH it can predict progression, provide an
estimate of prostate volume and guide
treatment

✧ If a patient has a strong family history of
prostate cancer he can use regular screening
PSA tests to permit early detection of the
disease.

Cons of a PSA test

✧ False positives (especially borderline values)
can lead to having a biopsy when there is
no cancer present with the risks of bleeding
and infection

✧ Anxiety of waiting for results

✧ If a patient does have cancer, PSA alone
cannot predict if this is likely to cause them
problems in the future

✧ A normal PSA does not categorically exclude
the presence of prostate cancer

✧ Very small cancers may be detected which
carry a very low risk of progression (see
explanation below) and may not need
treatment.

The percentage of men with prostate cancer rises
as the population studied becomes older. We
now know that many men do have a small area
of cancer in their prostate gland but this does not
result in any symptoms or problems in their
natural lifetimes. That is to say they can expect
to die *with* an undetected prostate cancer not
from it.

The anxiety caused by knowing of the presence
of a small cancer might reduce a man's quality of
life through unnecessary worry, whereas, it could
be argued that ignorance is bliss. In this situation
it is necessary to take into account the anger a
man may feel when the chance of an early

diagnosis is missed. However, fears of this sort of over-diagnosis have lessened as scientific research has shown that these small and insignificant cancers seldom result in a significantly raised PSA and a positive biopsy and anyway can be identified and managed by active surveillance, rather than immediate treatment.

PSA screening and the issues surrounding it

Prostate cancer screening involves offering *all* men above a certain age a regular PSA test, even though they have no symptoms, in order to detect prostate cancer at an early stage. This is quite different from a doctor suggesting a PSA test as part of his investigation of a patient who has come to consult him for a urological problem. At present, there is no national screening programme for prostate cancer in the UK using PSA. Nonetheless, the matter is under constant review by urologists, the government and the media. In 2002 the Department of Health modified its policy on PSA testing and has agreed that men are entitled to have a PSA test once they have received sufficient information to make an informed choice.

A screening programme is justified only if the screening test is accurate and effective treatment is available. Unfortunately, the PSA test, as we have just discussed, is not completely accurate at diagnosing cancer and requires the patient to go on to have prostate biopsies that are invasive, uncomfortable and carry a modest risk of bleeding and urine infections. Furthermore, studies have yet to prove conclusively that screening the population with the aim of detecting early prostate cancers will reduce the number of men who die of the disease as compared to the status quo. However, there is

organ-confined disease

A prostate cancer that is buried within the prostate gland with no spread outside of it. This means that if the prostate gland is removed during surgery or destroyed by radiation the cancer can be cured.

much work being done in this field with increasingly encouraging results that regular PSA testing in men does result in more prostate cancers being detected while they are still **organ-confined** and therefore suitable for potentially curative treatment. Other tests, such as the UPM3 urine based test (sometimes called the PCA3 test), which looks for specific genetic changes which occur in prostate cancer cells, may eventually replace PSA testing.

This is not to say that just because the present balance of opinion is that a national screening programme should not be instituted, that this will never be the case. There is much ongoing research into ways to enhance the accuracy of the PSA test to improve its usefulness as a screening tool and to strengthen the pro-screening cause. Furthermore, emerging work from USA and Europe would seem to indicate that screening PSA in younger men, i.e. those between 50 and 60 years, could give a survival benefit. This is thought to be because this group of men tends to develop more aggressive prostate cancers and they also have between 15 and 25 years remaining life expectancy. There are large-scale long-term studies with many thousands of men participating – the results of which should be available towards the end of this decade we hope it will clarify whether or not state sponsored screening for all men say between 60 and 65, using PSA should be introduced.

CHAPTER

6 Treatment of cancer confined to the prostate gland

When a man has been diagnosed with prostate cancer and the aggressiveness (grade) and degree of spread (stage) has been assessed, he will usually return to see his specialist team to discuss treatment options, often accompanied by his family or supporters. This is an important consultation and the man with prostate cancer should feel free to bring along with him anyone he likes to offer support and to be an 'extra set of ears'. There is often a lot of information to absorb so a pen and notepad, or even a tape recorder, can also come in handy. The patient and relatives should not be afraid to ask the specialist to fully explain the treatment proposed and should not be afraid to ask questions or for further explanations. It might take more than one visit to come to a decision and because prostate cancer is often slow growing (frequently estimated to double in size every two to three years) minor delays to seldom matter. Also, the patient should take the time to look at some of the very informative charity websites listed in

myth
The treatment of prostate cancer should be started as soon as possible.

fact
Prostate cancer, unlike some other cancers, is slow growing, doubling in size every two to three years. Treatment can therefore be delayed for quite some time while the specialist and man with prostate cancer work out the best way to take the treatment forward.

'Further help' (page 133) and to talk to a nurse counsellor.

This chapter examines the treatment options for those men whose prostate cancer has not spread beyond the prostate gland. These men are in the fortunate position of their cancer being potentially curable. As the cancer is localized in a small area, the treatment can be targeted at destroying the prostate gland and the cancer it contains, thus stopping it from spreading. However, no two men, or their cancers, are the same and each treatment given results from many different factors being considered. This is why it is important that the man with the disease fully understands the reasoning behind his treatment and agrees it is the preferred choice for him and for his family. He must also be prepared to accept that there are risks (for example, problems with erections and risks of incontinence or bowel disturbance) as well as benefits associated with all of the treatment options.

Active surveillance

As clinicians we aim to treat the whole person, not just the cancer that is inside the patient. If you consider two men, one aged 54 and the other 84, with cancer confined to the prostate, the treatment advised will often be different. This is because the overall health of these two men is not going to be the same. The 84-year-old may have other serious medical conditions and a life expectancy of less than ten years, so an 'aggressive' treatment, such as surgery, needs to be considered very carefully. Some of the surgical and radiotherapy treatments described below can cause side effects, especially in the short term. It might therefore be the case that a man and his family decide not to go for an active treatment but hope that the man will die naturally *with* his prostate cancer not *from* it, having enjoyed his final years to the full.

> **Q How likely is it that I will suffer from erection problems or incontinence after surgery?**
>
> **A** To a degree this depends on the experience of the surgeon operating on you and you should ask them for their own figures. Accepted pooled international figures are that 30–70 per cent of men will suffer erection problems and 2–15 per cent will suffer from some incontinence.

Conversely there are some younger men who decide that they do not want to risk the side effects of treatment, especially the risks to potency and continence, as they feel young and fit. Again, because the prostate cancer is slow growing, treatment could be delayed until a time when the patient is happy to go ahead. There is one problem with this strategy – once the prostate cancer has spread outside of the prostate gland the chances of cure drop significantly.

Active surveillance (which is a more proactive form of watchful waiting), as the name suggests, involves regular check-ups but no specific medical or surgical treatment. Most patients will be reviewed every four to six months to make sure there are no new developments and the man is not experiencing any problems. Regular PSA tests and clinical examinations are undertaken. If the PSA starts to rise or there is increasing pain or difficulty passing urine the situation will be re-assessed, biopsies sometimes repeated and treatment started where indicated.

If a man chooses the active surveillance option, he must, for his own peace of mind, be

active surveillance
This is when a man is monitored closely and his symptoms controlled but no treatment is given to the prostate cancer. It is aimed at keeping quality of life high and is frequently used in older men or those with medical conditions that would limit their life expectancy.

convinced that it is the right decision for him. The whole point of active surveillance is that the quality of life remains good – if he starts to worry, perhaps waking up in the night with anxiety attacks, his quality of life is suffering. If this happens the specialist or GP will want to know about it because it could be that alternative treatments will be better suited in this case. Many men, and their families, also find that becoming involved with a support group or charity helps. Talking to other men who are being treated in the same way can be very helpful.

Survival

The likelihood that the cancer will spread depends to a large extent on how aggressive it is. For men whose cancer shows a Gleason score of less than 7, the ten-year survival rate is around 87 per cent (this means that, after ten years, 87 men in 100 will not have died from prostate cancer; conversely, 13 men in 100 will have died from their prostate cancer). With more aggressive cancers (those with Gleason scores of 7 or above), the survival rate drops considerably (the ten-year survival rate for men with poorly-differentiated tumours has been calculated at an average of only 26 per cent).

Radical prostatectomy

lymph nodes
These occur at regular intervals throughout the lymphatic system and act as small filters, so cells such as cancer cells tend to accumulate at these points. The swollen glands you get in your neck during the flu are an example of lymph nodes.

Radical prostatectomy involves the surgical removal of the whole prostate gland along with the associated seminal vesicles and usually the nearby **lymph nodes** at time of surgery. The main advantage of performing this surgery is that if the prostate cancer is localized to the prostate gland there is no better way of being completely and demonstrably cured. The reason why not every man who has organ-confined prostate cancer undergoes this operation is that there are some significant side effects, namely **incontinence** and **impotence**, and the surgery itself is not always a breeze. If a man is to have a radical prostatectomy he needs to be medically fit and physically strong enough to handle it. He also needs to be in the hands of an experienced team who can deal with any situation that may arise.

Who should have a radical prostatectomy?

Again it must be stressed that no two men are the same and the following are widely accepted, but not cast-iron, guidelines that are used in the treatment decisions. As mentioned above a radical prostatectomy is probably the best way to cure prostate cancer, but is only effective if the cancer is still confined within the prostate gland. There is little point in removing a prostate gland at an operation, only to leave some cancer behind in the body. Unfortunately, once the cancer has breached the surrounding prostate capsule, there will sometimes be small deposits of cancer cells left behind. Therefore only men without evidence of prostate cancer outside of the gland will be offered this surgery. This information comes from the clinical findings including the PSA value and biopsy results plus sometimes MRI and bone scans.

The other main prerequisite is that the man is young enough and fit enough to benefit from being put through the surgery. Bluntly put, this usually means men younger than 70 years, as they have on average more than ten years' life expectancy. If a man with prostate cancer has another major medical problem, especially heart or breathing problems, they may be advised against an operation even though they are not

incontinence
The uncontrolled leakage of urine at any time other than when you urinate. It can be a small amount due to a weakness in the sphincter or complete loss of control if the sphincter is badly damaged.

impotence
This is when there is a problem in gaining an erection or one strong enough for penetrative intercourse.

myth
The specialist will decide how to treat my prostate cancer.

fact
The treatment of prostate cancer is a joint decision between the patient and his specialist. As the treatment options can include side-effects, such as incontinence and impotence, the man with prostate cancer should take an active interest in his treatment.

yet 70. There are two reasons for this: their medical condition might have already shortened their life expectancy and their problem may also make the physical risks of the surgery too great. In these men there is evidence from various studies to suggest that less demanding irradiation therapy will allow them to survive just as long as surgery.

Finally, as with all the options we are going to discuss, there is patient choice. In many cases it is difficult to categorically say which treatment is going to allow that man to live the longest. There will be unsuitable options that the specialist will advise against. Of the rest, the specialist team will discuss the advantages and disadvantages with the patient, his partner and supporters and see what they feel. For example, with radical prostatectomy, some men are attracted to the idea of the prostate and the cancer being physically removed from their body, but others will categorically not want to undergo surgery.

How a radical prostatectomy is done

The operation usually takes between two and three hours and the man can expect to stay in hospital between four and seven days.

An open radical prostatectomy is usually performed under a general anaesthetic so the patient will have no recollection of the operation itself. Specialist doctors called anaesthetists are responsible for putting people to sleep temporarily and supporting their bodily functions while the operation is being done. Anaesthetists also have a very important role in preventing and controlling pain in the period immediately after the operation, which is addressed in more detail below. The anaesthetist will usually see the patient either the night before or on the day of the operation and ask some general questions about health and lifestyle. He or she will then go through what will happen in the operating theatre, including how they will give the anaesthetic and what it will be like when the patient wakes up afterward. Often **epidural** or spinal anaesthetics, similar to those given to women in childbirth, are also given to help control discomfort immediately after the procedure. If this is planned then the anaesthetist will explain how this is done and why.

During the operation a cut will be made through the lower abdomen, either horizontally or vertically, just above the pubic bone, and the prostate and seminal vesicles will be removed. Samples from the lymph nodes nearest to the prostate will often also be taken to check whether the cancer has spread to these sites, which is now seldom the case. The so-called **cavernous nerves**, which are important for achieving an erection, are situated in bundles running to each side of the prostate. These nerves will be identified during the operation and the surgeon will take particular care not to disturb them (this may not be possible where the cancer has spread very close to the nerves); this is called a nerve-sparing approach which has been shown to enhance the recovery of potency after the operation.

The urethra, the tube that runs from the bladder through the prostate and down the penis, will have been cut just below the bladder neck and above the urethral sphincter that is important for continence. Once the prostate has been removed the cut end of urethra is then joined to the bladder, therefore reconstructing the tube that allows urine to exit from the bladder. While still under the anaesthetic a catheter will be inserted so that urination can continue while the join (technically called the **anastomosis**) between the bladder and urethra heals. A catheter is a soft silicone tube that runs down the

epidural
A technique an anaesthetist may use to control pain during and after an operation. An injection of local anaesthetic is put around the spinal cord to numb the body from that level down.

cavernous nerves
These are the nerves that initiate erections. The nerves run alongside the prostate gland and can be damaged during a radical prostatectomy.

anastomosis
The medical term for the joining back together of two cut ends of tube when a length has been removed at surgery. An anastomosis is performed in the urethra during a radical prostatectomy.

fact

Some men feel that the penis is a little shorter as the shortened urethra pulls back the penis. The circumference of the penis is not changed and when erect, men do not report much difference. With time the urethra often relaxes and the slight loss in length when the penis is flaccid disappears.

urethra from the bladder to the outside world. The catheter is prevented from falling out by inflating a balloon at the end of the catheter once inside the bladder. This balloon then can be deflated before the catheter is removed. The catheter will usually have to stay in place for around a fortnight. Once the catheter is removed the patient will be encouraged to perform pelvic floor exercises to help strengthen the urinary sphincter and help avoid incontinence that can be troublesome when the patient coughs, sneezes or stands up suddenly.

The hospital stay and post-operative recovery after open surgery

On waking from the surgery the patient is likely to have several tubes coming from him that were put in place while they were under anaesthetic. First, the catheter will be continuously draining urine from the bladder into a bag. The urine may look a little red for a couple of days, but the blood clears with time. Next there is likely to be one, or sometimes two, 'drain' tubes coming out through the wall of the lower abdomen. These drain bloody fluid from the site of the operation for the first 48 hours or so and help to prevent bruising. These drains are usually removed after the first couple of days. Finally there will be a drip giving clear fluid directly into a vein in the arm. Patients who have had a prostatectomy often don't feel like eating and drinking for a day or two and the drip prevents dehydration. Blood transfusion is now seldom necessary during or after radical prostatectomy, but blood is always available if it is required.

All patients who have had a radical prostatectomy are encouraged to get out of bed and sit in a chair and then to gently walk around as soon as possible. This reduces the risk of blood clots in the calves (deep vein thrombosis or 'DVT'), as does the use of heparin injections just beneath the skin, and means the patient can go home sooner. Most men will stay in hospital between four and six days. Patients will not be sent home unless they are walking, eating and drinking and are able to look after their catheter themselves.

Once at home, men who have had a radical prostatectomy find that they tire easily during recuperation. It may be necessary to take a nap during the day, which is fine, but men should resist the temptation to spend too much time in bed. Unless some exercise is taken each day then the body won't get stronger and recovery will be delayed. Most men will need six to eight weeks to convalesce and should not return to work for at least six weeks. Driving is not recommended for the first two to four weeks after surgery. The last piece of advice is that because of the cut in the muscles of the lower abdomen, men should not lift anything heavy for two weeks and should take things gently for a further eight to twelve weeks. Lifting heavy objects and straining can weaken the wound in the abdomen and lead to a hernia, an abnormal bulge of bowels through a weakened wound or through either groin.

Although most people feel they would not be able to look after a catheter, it is in fact very easy. During the day the catheter is attached to a long thin bag that can be strapped to the leg and hidden under clothes. At night this smaller capacity bag is swapped for a larger one to go by the bed so it does not need emptying overnight. Both types of bags have a simple tap that allows them to be emptied in a toilet. It is usual that the catheter placed at the operation remains for about two weeks, but some surgeons advise shorter or longer periods. If the catheter is dislodged or removed too early it can cause damage to the

myth
People will be able to tell you are wearing a catheter.

fact
This is not true, there are many people leading normal lives while wearing a catheter and no one knows that they have one. During the day a long thin leg bag can be strapped to the thigh to drain the catheter. Under a pair of trousers nobody will be able to see it. When the leg bag is full a tap at its base can be used to drain it directly into a toilet.

anastomosis (the join between the bladder and urethra) or damage the sphincter valve that maintains urinary continence. If the catheter becomes blocked and causes discomfort and pain due to an over-distended bladder, the patient should attend a hospital as soon as possible. If the urine becomes heavily blood stained, then drinking large amounts of fluid to produce lots of urine to flush the blood through is advised. Again, if bleeding is prolonged or very heavy and associated with the passage of clots the man with prostate cancer should return to the hospital where the problem can usually be easily resolved.

Newer ways of performing radical prostatectomies

Surgical technology is advancing at an ever-increasing pace and not surprisingly these new technologies are now being applied to the treatment of prostate cancer. Laparoscopy enables surgeons to work inside the body cavity through much smaller incisions and, although this can increase the operating time, it also reduces the hospital stay and enables the patient to get back to work quicker. Several units in the UK are now offering laparoscopic radical prostatectomies with good initial results. However, it remains to be seen whether or not this becomes the standard way to perform the procedure in the same way that it has in the case of the surgical removal of the gall bladder.

A further technological advance is the development of the so-called De Vinci™ robot that permits the surgeon to work with very great precision and spectacular magnification from a console which is remote from the patient. The entry ports are similar to those employed for a laparoscopic radical prostatectomy and the recovery time is quicker than the open surgical approach. It is still to be seen whether the results are better in terms of cancer cure, potency or rapid return of continence.

Follow-up

Naturally all men undergoing a radical prostatectomy are concerned and anxious that they will suffer from one of the two main side effects, namely incontinence and impotence. During the surgery all the tissues around the prostate become bruised and take a while to settle down and heal again. Impotence is due to damage to some of the nerves in the area immediately adjacent to the operative site and therefore erections will be absent or impaired immediately after surgery in all cases. Evaluation of strength of erections is not assessed until at least three months after surgery to give these nerves the chance to recover. If the erections are absent or not strong enough to have intercourse, then treatment options will be discussed at this point. There now are many treatments for this problem including tablets, pellets, injections directly into the penis or simply by talking through the problems and worries. Furthermore, as the impotence is due to surgery any treatment is available on an NHS prescription (see Chapter 12). Severe problems with incontinence are rare, and also tend to improve with time. If after a year there is still significant leakage the reason may be that the sphincter mechanism is damaged and will need consideration for repair with an artificial sphincter. Nevertheless, a significant proportion of men will leak a little urine on coughing, sneezing or standing up suddenly, immediately post operatively, especially if they have a full bladder. This is because the muscle of the sphincter has become weak and, just like any muscle, responds to exercise. The exercises are pelvic floor exercises and are the same as the ones taught to women who leak urine after childbirth. Also, like any other exercise, the benefits last only as long as you keep it up so the pelvic floor exercises need to be done regularly (ideally every hour) for maximum effect.

After the operation, the PSA level will be monitored as a way of gauging how successful the operation has been (see Figure 6.1).

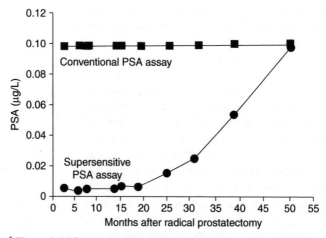

Figure 6.1 PSA recurrence after radical prostatectomy: supersensitive assays will reveal recurrence earlier.

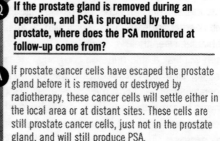

Q **If the prostate gland is removed during an operation, and PSA is produced by the prostate, where does the PSA monitored at follow-up come from?**

A If prostate cancer cells have escaped the prostate gland before it is removed or destroyed by radiotherapy, these cancer cells will settle either in the local area or at distant sites. These cells are still prostate cancer cells, just not in the prostate gland, and will still produce PSA.

The PSA will have already dropped by the time the catheter comes out at two weeks, but the PSA does not settle to its lowest reading until about three months after the operation. If the operation has been successful, it should remain almost undetectable indefinitely (usually reported as a level of less than 0.1 ng/ml on modern PSA analysis machines). Unfortunately, in up to one-third of men who have a radical prostatectomy, small deposits of the cancer will already have spread outside of the prostate and hence will not have been removed. If this is the case and the PSA level remains slightly elevated and/or starts to rise during follow-up, your doctor may recommend a 'mop-up' course of radiotherapy or alternatively some medicine. The PSA level will usually be checked every three to six months. As long as it stays low, no further action will be taken. If the PSA starts to increase rapidly or there is a sustained prolonged increase then the specialist team may want to double check that secondary deposits of prostate cancer are not present. This will usually entail repeating some scans and sometimes performing another biopsy. In general, the longer the interval between the original operation and the subsequent rise in the PSA, the better the outlook. In most cases a rising PSA after radical prostatectomy can be controlled by a course of radiotherapy which is given over a six- or seven-week period. Side effects of treatment include irritation of the rectum resulting in frequent bowel actions with some bleeding. This usually settles in time.

Possible side effects and risks

In experienced hands there is now only a small (less than 3 per cent) risk of persistent incontinence, but more than a 50 per cent chance of impotence following radical prostatectomy, at least initially. However, the risks of impotence can now be reduced by nerve-sparing techniques and can be treated effectively with both oral drugs and injection therapy in most cases. In both these situations your specialist will usually wait several months before initiating any long-term treatment as it can take this long for full erectile or sphincter function to return following the operation. There is some blood loss during the operation and approximately one in five men will require a minor blood transfusion, usually during the first few days. Finally, as the anastomosis (the join between the bladder and the urethra) heals it may narrow, causing difficulty in urinating, usually in the form of a poor stream and difficulty getting going. This happens in less than 10 per cent of men and is generally treated by dilating the narrowing under a brief general anaesthetic. This usually resolves the problem completely, although recurrence of the problem may sometimes occur, requiring a further stretch of the bladder neck.

The chance of side effects and the likely success of the operation are governed largely by the expertise of the urologist and his or her team. If you are offered this operation, ask your urologist:

✧ How many radical prostatectomy operations he or she has performed?
✧ What the results were from these operations?
✧ Whether he or she will be performing your surgery personally?
✧ What other team back-up is available?
✧ What are the arrangements for follow-up?

Survival

More than 80 per cent of men who have this operation are still alive ten years afterwards, and more than 60 per cent are still alive after 15 years. A recent study from North America, which followed men after radical prostatectomy, has shown that 82 per cent are disease free at 15 years. In a randomized study from Scandinavia, men with localized prostate cancer were allocated to either watchful waiting or radical prostatectomy. In the radical prostatectomy group the rate of developing cancer spread to the bone (metastases) was half that of those who had watchful waiting as therapy (Figure 6.2) and the chances of survival were significantly improved.

As a consequence many urologists feel that a radical prostatectomy is the treatment option most likely to offer a permanent cure for cancer confined to the prostate gland and with a Gleason score of 7 or less.

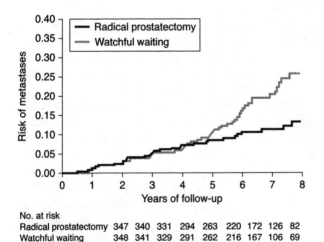

Figure 6.2 Radical prostatectomy versus watchful waiting.

Radiotherapy treatment

Radiotherapy treatment is the use of radiation in the form of gamma rays to destroy cells. The cell-killing effects of radiation were discovered in the 1930s. However, the usefulness of

linear accelerator
This is a machine that allows the focused delivery of radiation to the prostate gland. It looks a bit like an X-ray machine and the patient lies on a table in the middle of the machine to receive his treatment.

radiotherapy
The use of radiation to kill cancer cells. With external beam radiotherapy the radiation is generated from an external source and focused on to the prostate.

brachytherapy
A type of radiotherapy that uses radioactive pellets implanted directly into the prostate gland.

radiotherapy in prostate cancer was hampered as it was difficult to get a sufficient dose of radiation to the prostate which is located deep inside the body. The advent of a machine called a **linear accelerator** revolutionized this form of treatment. This discovery allowed beams of strong gamma radiation to be targeted to a defined area within the body and hence made prostate irradiation possible. Nowadays radiation treatment is delivered in two main ways: external beam **radiotherapy** in which beams of radiation are shone from outside the body and targeted on the prostate; alternatively, **brachytherapy**, literally 'short treatment', where tiny radioactive seeds or beads are placed directly in the prostate so they irradiate the gland from the inside out.

Who should have radiotherapy?

It is sometimes thought that the men who have radiotherapy are negatively selected, that is they were unsuitable for a prostate surgery. However, radiotherapy is certainly not a second best option. If a man is too frail to be considered for surgery, radiotherapy can still be a potentially curative treatment. Therefore, those men who have medical conditions that make surgery less than ideal should be considered for radiotherapy. Medical evidence also suggests that radiotherapy is better than surgery for the very aggressive cancers (Gleason score 8 and above) as the radiotherapy is particularly effective in eradicating these rapidly growing cells. These very aggressive cancers are also more likely to have small breaches of the prostate capsule, which are not detectable even with the best scanners. This is where the second real advantage of radiotherapy becomes apparent; the area immediately around the prostate can be included in the radiation zone and hence treated.

Studies have also shown that some men with a high risk of recurrent cancer may benefit first from brachytherapy (see page 73), followed by a short dose of external beam radiotherapy afterward. This group of men comprises those with a locally advanced cancer and a PSA higher than 10 ng/ml or a Gleason score between 8 and 10.

However, there are some men for whom radiotherapy is not ideal. These are the men with large prostate glands that are obstructing bladder emptying or causing a very diminished urinary steam. As the radiation kills the prostate cells the gland initially swells before shrivelling up. Obviously, if a man has problems urinating before his treatment they will worsen for the first couple of months following treatment. This can result in a complete cessation of bladder emptying – urinary retention. Because of the temporary swelling caused by the insertion of the radioactive seeds, brachytherapy is especially likely to cause this in men with pre-existing prostatic obstruction.

Radiotherapy can be planned as the treatment once the patient's wishes and those of his family are taken into account. Some men prefer to avoid surgery, catheterization or hospital stays. If a patient has strong views, these should be communicated to his specialist team. In contrast to surgery, external beam radiotherapy is an outpatient treatment requiring minimal hospital stays. It is important that the patient is involved in the decision making process and feels reassured that the treatment is the best option for them.

How is external beam radiotherapy done?

The first step in this treatment is careful planning – the gamma rays need to be accurately targeted and the correct dose used so that they reach the prostate gland. Furthermore, the radiation needs to be delivered to the same spot for many consecutive sessions and therefore positioning is very important.

The patient will be invited to attend the radiotherapy department for planning which can take some time. First, a CT scan is performed so that an accurate idea of the size and shape of the prostate gland, the target, is gained. The surrounding organs such as the bladder above and the bowel behind are also noted as well as the dimensions of the pelvis and thickness of the abdominal wall. In some departments specialist computers are used to make virtual three-dimensional reconstructions of the pelvis to help keep the area exposed to the radiotherapy limited to that containing prostate cancer and not the surrounding healthy tissue.

Next, specialized technicians calculate the strength of radiation beam needed to penetrate the prostate gland, but not pass through it and into the bowel behind. This can vary from man to man. The shape of the radiation beam is 'moulded' to prevent too many surrounding healthy areas being exposed. All the personalized settings are put into the radiotherapy machine so that exactly the same treatment protocol is followed every time. Finally the patient will have small blue dots tattooed on to his skin to act as alignment markers so that when he lies on the treatment couch for 15 to 20 minutes each day the machine is always pointing at the same spot. Once the planning is complete, the treatments themselves can be delivered quickly, while safe in the knowledge that the same area will receive the correct dose of radiation each and every time. The latest radiotherapy machines deliver what is known as 'conformal' radiotherapy – this is precise targeted treatment (see Figure 6.3). You should ask your radiation oncologist whether the radiotherapy machines he or she will use can deliver conformal treatment.

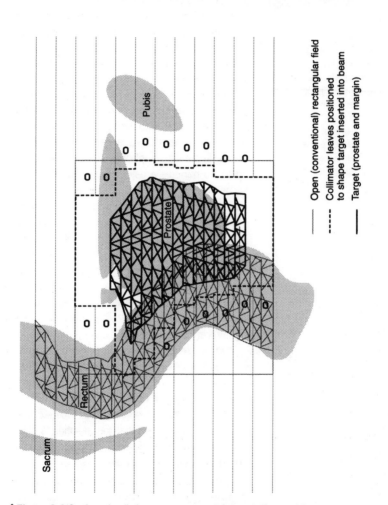

Sacrum

Rectum

Prostate

Pubis

—— Open (conventional) rectangular field

---- Collimator leaves positioned
     to shape target inserted into beam

—— Target (prostate and margin)

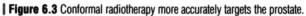

Figure 6.3 Conformal radiotherapy more accurately targets the prostate.

fact
Wrong, it is remarkably painless. The skin that the radiation beam goes through will feel warm and look a little red immediately after the treatment, a little like after sitting out in the sun. Most men find the biggest problem with external beam radiation is feeling tired as well as bladder and bowel upsets.

The treatments themselves are much simpler. The patient will need to come to the radiotherapy department every weekday, Monday to Friday, to have radiotherapy. Everyone has a break at the weekend. The patient will lie flat on his back or stomach on the table with the radiotherapy machine around him. The machine is a little like an X-ray machine with large arms usually above and to the sides of the table. As the treatment is given there may be some movement of the arms of the machine around the patient. All the patient has to do is lie still. As a general rule people do not find it claustrophobic. The treatment lasts up to 20 minutes a day and the patient can go home straight afterwards. Towards the end of the six-week treatment many patients complain of tiredness and lower bowel symptoms including urgency and rectal bleeding. Recently a study in the USA has shown that rectal cancers are slightly more common after external beam radiotherapy. If rectal bleeding occurs months or years after previous radiation treatment to the prostate then further investigations should be undertaken to exclude this.

Studies have shown that three months of hormone treatment given before the radiotherapy has improved the long-term survival of patients and is now widely used. It is thought that the hormone treatment shrinks the prostate and the cancer within it, so that the radiation is more likely to 'hit' the cancer cells, which are now concentrated in a smaller area.

Follow-up

In some ways this is similar to surgery: regular trips to the specialist with PSA blood tests to monitor any relapse of the cancer. Radiotherapy destroys a cell by disrupting its DNA – the material that controls cell division – and hence causing it to die the next time it tries to grow or repair itself. As a result there is a time lag between receiving the radiotherapy and the prostate cancer being destroyed. Because of this there is a longer period of time, compared to surgery, before the PSA value falls. It is not unusual to wait three months before the PSA is measured for the first time to gauge a response. In most cases the PSA drops to a figure below 1.0 ng/ml but each man is different and the PSA value may bottom out a little higher. What is important over time is the overall trend. If the PSA is steadily rising with time, especially if it is doubling in less than a year, this could be an indication to look for further prostate cancer locally or distant deposits (metastases). If this is the case then there will be further discussion about what to do next. Options such as hormone therapy, active surveillance or cryotherapy (freezing the gland) can all be considered to control the recurrent disease (see later in this Chapter and Chapter 7 for more information).

Possible side effects and risks

Most men undergoing radiotherapy will find it tiring. This tends to be a cumulative effect with the patient feeling more fatigued towards the end of the treatment. The weekends off are often a good time to rest up and recuperate. If travelling to and from the radiotherapy department is becoming difficult, feel free to discuss it with someone in the department as help with transport or moving to a more convenient time slot can usually be arranged to make the treatment as easy as possible.

The main side effect is a need to urinate more often, sometimes with a strong feeling of urgency and sometimes urinary incontinence. This effect is usually mild and is due to the nearby radiation irritating the bladder. Unfortunately, despite the best efforts to protect nearby healthy tissue a very small proportion of men (less than 2–3 per cent) will be severely affected. If this is the case, a rest from radiotherapy can settle the symptoms.

There can also be irritation or discomfort around the rectum, sometimes accompanied by diarrhoea and bleeding. Again, this side effect is usually temporary, lasting only for a few weeks while the radiotherapy is being given. Very occasionally, the rectal injury is disabling, with bleeding, altered bowel habit and pain, making a colostomy necessary. A colostomy is a diversion of the bowel so that the bowel content is drained into a sealed stoma bag stuck to the skin of the abdomen. This is discreet, odourless and very rarely leaks. As mentioned above, recent information suggests that radiation to the prostate slightly increases the risk of rectal cancer. Persistent rectal bleeding after external beam radiotherapy should always be investigated.

Finally, just like surgery, men can suffer form erection problems. Between 20 and 30 per cent of men who have undergone radiotherapy will develop problems with their erections as a direct result. This problem tends to develop gradually, over 6 to 18 months, and can usually be overcome with the use of oral or alternative treatments that can be prescribed by the doctor.

Survival

At best, the survival rates with radiotherapy are comparable with those associated with radical prostatectomy. Several published studies have put the 15-year survival rates at 40–60 per cent (that is, between 40 and 60 men out of 100 will still be alive after 15 years).

Brachytherapy

As mentioned above, brachytherapy is a special form of radiation treatment for prostate cancer. In brachytherapy, instead of the radiation being targeted to the prostate from outside in, the radiation is placed directly into the prostate gland itself. However, both brachytherapy and external beam radiotherapy are using the same science, that radiation disrupts the DNA in a cell's nucleus and causes it to self-destruct the next time it tries to grow or repair itself.

Brachytherapy is still a relatively new technique in the UK and not all hospitals have the specialist equipment or people with the skills to implant the radioactive seeds into the prostate precisely. If the patient has a particular interest in discussing brachytherapy, and his specialist feels that this could be a beneficial treatment for him, they will arrange an appointment in the nearest unit.

How is brachytherapy done?

The procedure involves the implantation of between 60 and 100 radioactive seeds, depending on the size of the gland, into the prostate. The most common material for the seeds to be made of is Iodine-125 or, less commonly, a substance called Palladium-103. The seeds are then left inside the patient where they gradually lose their radioactivity (decay) over the following 12 months or so. The seeds are not removed from the prostate even once they have completely lost all the beneficial radiation. They are quite safe to be left in the prostate in the long term and their position can be checked easily with a simple X-ray or CT scan. Occasionally, a brachytherapy seed can migrate through the bloodstream to the lung or elsewhere. If this occurs it can be diagnosed on an X-ray, but in practice it doesn't seem to cause any trouble.

Prior to the procedure, the dose of radiotherapy and position of the seeds are carefully worked out so that it is as effective and accurate as possible in killing the prostate cancer. The brachytherapy procedure is usually performed under a spinal or light general anaesthetic. The patient is positioned on their back with the legs apart and raised in special stirrups; similar to the position used in gynaecological procedures. This allows easy access to the back passage and the perineum (the area behind the scrotum and in front of the anus). First, a thin ultrasound probe will be inserted into the rectum so that the surgeon and radiation specialist can see images of the prostate. Then, using the ultrasound image as a guide, hollow needles are inserted through the skin between the scrotum and back passage into the prostate, which sits deeper in the pelvis above the perineum. The radioactive seeds are then placed in the prostate by pushing them down the hollow needles, which in turn are withdrawn. The ultrasound image is used throughout the procedure to watch the insertion and check the position of the seeds (see Figure 6.4). A catheter will be inserted to help pass urine after the operation. The catheter might need to stay in place for a couple of days, but patients can normally go home without a catheter within 24 hours.

Most patients feel somewhat bruised down below following brachytherapy but this soon settles. There is a high chance that bruises will occur across the perineum but bruising in the scrotum or penis is rare. On discharge from the hospital, painkillers will be given to control the discomfort and it is advised that the patient sits on a pillow for a day or two! Alpha blocking medicine, such as Flomax™ (tamsulosin) can be helpful in improving any restriction of urinary flow which is not uncommon for several months after brachytherapy.

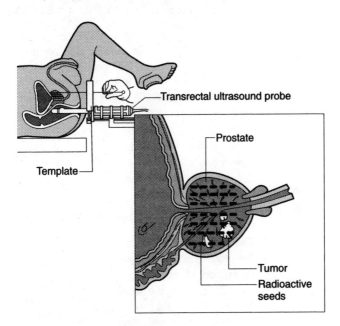

Transrectal ultrasound probe

Prostate

Template

Tumor

Radioactive seeds

Figure 6.4 Brachytherapy involves implantation of radioactive seeds into the prostate.

Side effects and risks

As the radiation is being targeted at the prostate so accurately, incontinence and rectal damage tend to be less common after brachytherapy than after external beam. Nevertheless, the impotency rates are broadly similar to conventional external beam radiotherapy with erection difficulties developing over the months following the treatment, but these do usually respond to treatment. For the first few weeks after brachytherapy the prostate swells in response to the treatment. Not surprisingly, therefore, many patients complain of a reduced urinary flow and some frequency of passing urine.

Survival and outcomes

The results of brachytherapy are not as well documented as those of radical prostatectomy as it is a newer treatment option. The longest follow-up is from Seattle where ten-year data are now available and the results look encouraging. More and more centres in the UK are now beginning to offer brachytherapy and it seems likely that, as has happened in the USA, this form of treatment is likely to become more and more popular because it avoids the obvious disadvantages of major surgery and the inconvenience of having to attend daily for six weeks of external beam radiotherapy.

Cryoablation of the prostate

This evolving technique freezes and then thaws the prostate cells twice over to bring about the destruction of cancer. Ice crystals form inside the cells disrupting the internal structures, and the freezing and thawing process puts huge stress on the membrane surrounding and containing the cells, which ruptures, killing the cells.

How is cryotherapy performed?

The procedure is performed under a spinal or light general anaesthetic, again with the patient on his back with legs up in stirrups. Specially designed needles are inserted into the prostate, under ultrasound guidance, through the perineum in a similar way to brachytherapy needles (see Figure 6.5).

Cryotherapy needles (or cryoprobes) circulate Argon gas through them which causes an 'ice ball' to form at the tip which overlaps with the ice ball formed by adjacent cryoprobes (see Figure 6.6). The quantity of circulating Argon can be altered so the size of the ice ball can be controlled and the total area frozen can be sculpted. During the procedure the prostate will be frozen and thawed twice over to destroy the prostate cancer cells. As it is important to avoid damage to the urethra, the tube running through the prostate draining the bladder, a special warming catheter, is used throughout the process. After the procedure a catheter will be left in for 7 to 14 days as, again, this treatment causes initial swelling of the prostate gland.

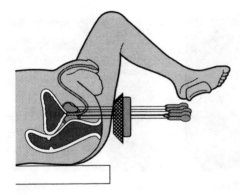

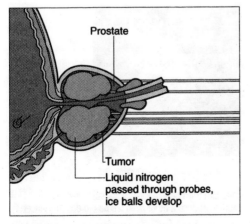

Prostate

Tumor

Liquid nitrogen passed through probes, ice balls develop

Figure 6.5 Cryotherapy aims to destroy cancer cells by freezing with cryotherapy needles.

Possible side effects and risks

The main risks are that the freezing process will damage the urethra or rectum. To reduce this risk a warmed catheter is placed in the urethra and warming probes placed near the rectal wall during the procedure. Permanent damage to the rectum is rare but fistulae have been reported. The largest study of cryotherapy side effects quotes incontinence rates at 4 per cent and impotence at 95 per cent with rectal damage being unusual.

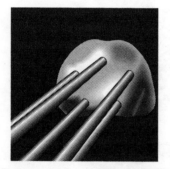

First generation – 3–8 mm probe, liquid

Second generation – 3,4 mm probe, gas

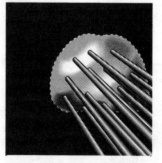

Third generation – cryoneedle, gas

Figure 6.6 First, second and third generation cryotherapy needles. The third generation probes produce a more even ice ball to destroy cancer within the prostate.

Most patients find that there is initial bladder irritation, in the form of urgency and frequency, but this usually settles with time.

Survival

This is still a relatively new technique but patients who have undergone this treatment have been followed up for nearly five years and some centres are showing disease free rates comparable with patients five years after having a radical prostatectomy or radiotherapy. This technique is of particular interest as it can be used to treat men in whom prostate cancer returns after a course of radiotherapy, when previously no potentially curative treatments were readily available.

High intensity focused ultrasound

This is the newest treatment for localized prostate cancer that is becoming more widely accepted. In high intensity focused ultrasound (HIFU), as the name suggests, concentrated ultrasound waves are focused on the prostate gland to destroy the prostate cells. The procedure can take up to two hours to complete and is performed under a general anaesthetic. A catheter is put in place at the time of the procedure and is retained for some days after because the prostate may swell in response to the therapy, making the normal passage of urine difficult. One appeal of this new treatment option is that it can be repeated without difficulty. However, as yet HIFU is relatively untested as a reliable means of destroying all cancer cells and is only available in very few centres.

my experience

I am a 56-year-old fireman and read about High Intensity Focused Ultrasound (HIFU) in my newspaper after having been recently diagnosed with prostate cancer on the basis of an elevated PSA of 4.8 ng/ml and a TRUS biopsy. I sought a specialist opinion and underwent treatment as part of a research protocol. The procedure took two hours and I needed to have a catheter for a week afterwards. My progress is still being followed up but I have normal erections and sexual function and my PSA has declined to 2.3 ng/ml. Further biopsies are planned to check that all the disease has been eradicated.

CHAPTER

7

Treatment of locally advanced or recurrent prostate cancer

If a man has prostate cancer that has spread beyond the capsule of the prostate and has invaded the surrounding tissues he is said to have a **locally advanced disease**. This is very different from distant spread of the cancer, for example into the bones or the liver, which is described as metastatic cancer and carries a much worse outlook. If we go back to the tumour-nodes-metastasis (TNM) grading system discussed in Chapter 4, men with locally advanced disease are described as stage T3 NO MO.

Men with locally advanced prostate cancer may face a difficult decision in deciding which treatment option to choose. Men in this category fall into a 'grey area' between curable organ-confined disease and incurable metastatic cancer. Which treatment is finally undertaken will depend on the grade (aggressiveness) of the cancer and just how far from the prostate the cancer has spread (the clinical stage). The patient's age, general health and wishes as well as the desires of his family and close friends will

> **locally advanced disease**
> Prostate cancer that has spread outside the surrounding capsule of the prostate gland but has not, as yet, spread to distant areas in the body through the bloodstream.

be important as well. It is easy to appreciate that a low-grade cancer with only a minor breach of the prostate capsule could potentially be cured. This is in contrast to a high-grade cancer with a large volume of local spread. Treatments of these cancers concentrate on preventing spread to distant sites, but will unfortunately seldom totally eradicate the cancer in and around the prostate itself.

This chapter discusses some of the common treatment options used in this situation. Again this is a interactive process, the man with prostate cancer and a member of the specialist team need to sit down and discuss the pros, cons and acceptability of the available treatments. Many of the treatments below will not apply to all patients and the specialist will explain which he or she feels are most suitable and why. If the man who is to receive the treatment doesn't understand something or finds some part of it unacceptable he must make this clear to the doctor treating him. As clinicians we are used to finding the 'best fit' treatment for each individual person. The cancer nurse specialist and the telephone helplines and websites of the cancer charities (see 'Further help', page 133) can also be very helpful in the decision making process. In the end, the individual patient's preference and the wishes of his family should always be paramount.

The treatment options that can be considered include:

✧ Active surveillance
✧ Hormone therapy by either drugs or orchidectomy (surgery)
✧ Surgical castration
✧ Intermittent hormone therapy
✧ Hormone therapy followed by radical prostatectomy or radiotherapy.

Active surveillance

The rationale behind this approach has been outlined in the previous chapter and remains the same in this situation. Active surveillance (proactive watchful waiting) requires regular check-ups with PSA blood tests and possibly repeat biopsies. Treatment is targeted at controlling any symptoms, such as pain or difficulty passing urine.

Active surveillance in locally advanced prostate cancer is particularly suited to older men or those with other significant medical problems that are more likely than the prostate cancer itself to result in their death. The advantage of this approach includes the avoidance of the side effects of treatment which means that the patient gets the maximum quality out of his remaining years. It is important to realize, however, that at this stage, because the cancer is more advanced, it is much more likely to cause symptoms and to become life-threatening more quickly than a low-grade cancer that is still confined to the prostate.

Hormone therapy

When doctors talk about **hormone therapy** in the context of prostate cancer they are referring to depriving the prostate cancer of a specific hormone called testosterone. In the presence of normal levels of testosterone the prostate cancer is stimulated to grow and spread to other sites. Therefore, if the amount of testosterone in the body is reduced, prostate cancer growth can be slowed and the spread to the bones delayed or prevented. Hormone treatment won't kill all the cancer, but rather puts it into a form of 'hibernation', so the man can get on with living his life. Unfortunately, eventually the prostate cancer will usually start growing and spreading again despite the hormone treatment at which

hormone therapy
The use of drugs to block the stimulatory effects of testosterone on the growth of the prostate tissue and hence slow down the spread of prostate cancer.

hormone relapsed prostate cancer (HRPC)
A prostate cancer that has started to grow and spread again after a period of control with hormone therapy.

androgens
These are the hormones, or chemical messengers, that are particularly linked to the male sexual characteristics and organs. The most well known of the androgens is testosterone.

myth
Hormone treatment will turn me into a woman.

fact
While hormone treatment does reduce the levels of the main male hormone, testosterone, the feminizing effects of this are minimal. There are no changes in the pitch of the voice or in the figure. Some men notice that they do not have to shave as often and that the skin is softer, furthermore, hormone treatment can give hot flushes.

point it is called **hormone relapsed prostate cancer** or HRPC.

How hormone treatment works and why it eventually fails

Way back in the eighteenth century a famous Englishman, John Hunter (one of the founding fathers of modern surgery), documented that if you remove an animal's testicles (castration) their sex organs, including the prostate, shrank in size. It wasn't until the 1930s that the American scientists, Huggins and Hodges worked out that removing the testicles of animals shut down the production of the male hormone testosterone – which is an **androgen**. They neatly demonstrated this fact by reversing the effects of castration with testosterone injections. This Nobel Prize winning research also showed that prostate cancer shrunk when testosterone was reduced and that a patient's condition improved dramatically in response to deprivation of testosterone (so-called androgen deprivation).

Over the last 80 years this has continued to be an area of intense interest generating huge amounts of research information. The reason for this is that reducing testosterone did not prove to be the total magic cure of prostate cancer. Unfortunately, with time, prostate cancer escapes the control of the hormone treatment and starts to grow and spread again. It is now understood that this is because prostate cancer has more than one type of prostate cancer cell. Within the cancer these different types of cells are all jumbled up together and do different things in the presence or absence of testosterone. They are divided into androgen-dependent cells and androgen-independent cells.

Androgen-dependent cancer cell types cannot survive in a low testosterone environment and these are the ones that are reduced by the hormone treatment. Unfortunately, there is a group of androgen-independent cells in the prostate cancer that are not affected by the level of testosterone in the system. These cells continue to divide regardless of what is happening to their androgen-dependent neighbours. At present there are few effective treatments for the androgen-independent cells, as they have a long lifespan and grow and divide slowly. This means that if conventional chemotherapy, as used in other types of cancer, is used against these cells they have time to repair any damage done and survive the chemotherapy attack. At present, however, there is a lot of exciting work being done to approach the problem from another angle, which is finding ways to stimulate these cells to die early. Of course, the trick to this is finding something that will only kill off the cancer cells and not affect other healthy cells in the body.

Types of hormone treatment available

Testosterone levels can be reduced through medication or surgery. The use of drugs has largely eclipsed **orchidectomy**, that is the surgical removal of the testicles, as the most common treatment, as the medications have become more efficient and acceptable to patients. In addition, medications can be stopped and started, while removal of the testicles is of course irreversible.

There are two main components to medical hormone treatment that can be given either individually, or in tandem. The first are luteinizing hormone releasing hormone (**LHRH**) **analogues**. LHRH is a naturally occurring hormone, and the analogue part of the name means that it is a synthetic form that has a structure similar to the natural form. The second

orchidectomy
The surgical removal of both testicles to reduce the amount of testosterone in the body. Orchidectomy is an irreversible form of hormone therapy.

LHRH analogues
Luteinizing hormone releasing hormone analogues are drugs that switch off the production of testosterone by the testicles. They are used in hormone therapy.

anti-androgens
Drugs which block the action of testosterone in the body and hence are also used in hormone therapy.

luteinizing hormone (LH)
This is produced by the brain and travels in the bloodstream to the testicles where it tells them to start producing testosterone.

are **anti-androgens**, which block the action of the male hormone testosterone in the body.

Although the testicles are the main producers of testosterone they are not just churning it out constantly from the day a man is born until his death. The brain, using a series of chemical messengers, or hormones, carefully controls production of testosterone. The process starts in an area of the brain that is responsible for regulating many of the body's hormones, called the hypothalamus. The hypothalamus produces pulses of LHRH that tells another area of the brain, called the pituitary, to release a substance called **luteinizing hormone** (**LH**). LH is the substance that drives the testicles to make testosterone. Once made by the testicles the testosterone enters the bloodstream and then diffuses into the cells of the prostate. This whole system is kept closely under control by the hypothalamus in the brain, which monitors the amount of testosterone in the bloodstream. If the testosterone level is too high the hypothalamus stops producing LHRH and therefore the testicles stop producing testosterone. This is called a feedback loop.

LHRH analogues

As the explanation above illustrates there are many steps in the process of the manufacture of testosterone by the testicles and this process can be stopped at several levels. The most commonly used drug to bring about chemical castration is the LHRH analogue. This substance works by tricking the pituitary gland into stopping production of LH. If the level of LH in the bloodstream drops the testicles stop making testosterone. Natural LHRH is produced in the hypothalamus and released in pulses. The pituitary detects these pulses of LHRH, which act as a Morse code, telling it to release LH to stimulate the testicles. The LHRH analogue used is a man-made version of LHRH with a similar chemical structure. The LHRH analogue once given is released as a constant stream, without any on and off pulses. In the first instance this over-stimulates the system causing an increase in the amount of testosterone, which may transiently stimulate the cancer. This is known as the **flare phenomenon**. After a period of about a week the pituitary gland becomes exhausted and simply stops producing the LH.

To protect patients from the effects of the temporary testosterone flare when started on LHRH analogues, they will often be given an anti-androgen for the first one or two weeks. Anti-androgens block the effects of testosterone on all the cells in the body that have androgen receptors which includes prostate cancer cells.

There are several main LHRH analogues on the market, including goserelin (Zoladex™) and leuprolide (Prostap™). Both of them are given as an injection, Zoladex under the skin and Prostap intramuscularly, in either monthly or three-monthly time intervals. This is usually done by the GP or district nurse, although in many areas the first dose of the LHRH analogue is given in a hospital outpatients' department following a few days of anti-androgen treatment.

Side effects

The main side effects of these drugs stem from the fact that they are reducing the body's testosterone (androgen) levels. Men will notice a reduction in their sex drive (libido) and lose the ability to achieve erections. These effects are reversible if the LHRH analogue is stopped, but will take some time to diminish. Hot flushes, similar to those women experience during their menopause, can be troublesome to some men.

flare phenomenon
When a man is first started on an LHRH analogue there is an initial surge in testosterone levels before they drop. To protect against stimulation of the prostate cancer during this period a short course of anti-androgens is given.

myth
Hot flushes are harmful.

fact
This is not the case. Some men find them inconvenient and troublesome but they do not do any long lasting damage.

It is impossible to predict who will be affected and how badly they will strike. They are not harmful to health, but many men find the sudden feeling of heat associated with sweating disconcerting and sometimes embarrassing.

Anti-androgens

These are compounds that make the prostate gland unresponsive to the testosterone in the bloodstream. The way a prostate cell picks up the signal from the testosterone is through a chemical receptor. In the prostate gland there are receptors that are unique to testosterone. Think of the receptor as a lock and testosterone the key that will turn within it. If you put the correct key in the lock it turns easily and activates the lock mechanism.

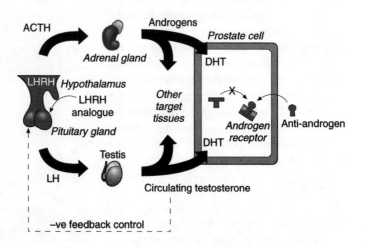

ACTH, adrenocorticotrophin hormone; DHT, dihydrotestosterone; LH, luteinizing hormone

Figure 7.1 The action of drugs which are used in prostate cancer.

Testosterone, when it comes near a testosterone receptor, will bind to it and set off a chain reaction inside that prostate cell. In the case of androgen sensitive prostate cancer cells this will stimulate them to grow and divide. However, other substances in the blood do not fit in the testosterone receptor and therefore do not trigger these effects. Anti-androgens are valuable medicines as they can fit into the receptor and then block it so that it is not available to detect testosterone. Think of it like a key that you can push into a lock but it is not quite the correct shape and therefore will not turn (see Figure 7.1).

There are several anti-androgens available; flutamide, bicalutamide and cyproterone acetate. They are given in tablet form and must be taken every day. When these anti-androgens were first used to treat cancer they were added to LHRH analogue treatment if the PSA was increasing. This became known as **maximal androgen blockade**, as together these medications both reduce testosterone production and the prostate's sensitivity to it. However, anti-androgens have now been shown to be just as effective as LHRH analogues or castration when used alone as long as there are no metastases present. A large international trial comparing once daily bicalutamide (Casodex™) to a placebo treatment showed that there was a 42 per cent reduction in the spread of cancer in men treated with the anti-androgen.

> **maximal androgen blockade**
> This is using LHRH analogues and anti-androgen at the same time to prevent a prostate cancer spreading.

Side effects

One of the main advantages of anti-androgens is that they do not reduce the levels of testosterone in the bloodstream. This means that men have a greater chance of preserving their sex drive and erections. For this reason anti-androgen treatment is becoming a popular choice among younger men with prostate cancer.

Anti-androgens can also sometimes give men stomach upsets and diarrhoea. On rare occasions anti-androgens can cause liver damage and therefore once the patient has been started on anti-androgens they should have regular blood tests to detect any change in liver function.

Surgical castration

Surgical castration (or bilateral orchidectomy) is the simplest and cheapest method to reduce a man's testosterone levels for good. It involves removing both testicles during a short surgical procedure and this brings about an irreversible drop in testosterone levels. This method of reducing testosterone is the most rapidly effective, with levels dropping by 90 per cent within hours of the operation.

The surgery itself can be performed either as day surgery or may require a night in hospital. Most men have a general anaesthetic so that they are unaware during the procedure. However, it can also be performed with a spinal anaesthetic, where the patient feels nothing from the waist down, or more rarely a local anaesthetic where an injection into the scrotum numbs the tissues before they are cut. A small cut is made in the scrotum. The blood vessels that supply the testicle and the vas deferens, the tube that carries the manufactured sperm back into the body prior to ejaculation, are tied and divided, then both testicles are removed. The scrotum is then sewn up again. So that the scrotum does not look empty some urologists will put in silicone plastic prosthetic testicles at the same time, if the patient wishes them. A dressing will be put over the scrotum to prevent excess bruising or post-operative bleeding and this can be removed the following day. Most patients are discharged within 24 hours.

Side effects

Men who opt for bilateral orchidectomy will have the same side effects as those receiving LHRH analogues. Their sex drive will reduce and they will lose their ability to achieve erections. It will also be impossible for them to father children. They may suffer from hot flushes as well. One of the main issues with orchidectomy is the psychological one. Men often feel scared that they will be 'feminized' by this procedure. Alteration in the tone of voice or development of more female features does not happen, but some men notice that they do not need to shave so frequently, that their skin texture softens and there is some loss of body hair.

As far as the operation is concerned, mild bruising of the scrotum is quite common, as is some discomfort for the first few days. Usually supportive underpants and simple painkillers will be sufficient to make the patient comfortable. More rarely a blood clot (haemotoma) can form inside the scrotum that will cause some pain over the 14–28 days it takes the body to reabsorb it, or an infection in the wound will require a short course of antibiotics to clear it up.

myth
The scrotum looks empty after orchidectomy.

fact
It is true that the scrotum will not look as full as it did when the testicles were there but many men are surprised that it is not as bad as they imagined. If this is something you feel strongly about then the surgeon can perform a procedure called a sub-capsular orchidectomy where more tissue is left behind to give bulk. Alternatively, silicone plastic testicles can be put in the scrotum for cosmetic effect.

Survival

Hormone therapy alone reduces the tumour size and slows the cancer progression in around 80 per cent of men with locally advanced disease. There is no great difference between the different types of medical hormone treatment and surgical methods. Remember that hormone therapy does not destroy all the cancer cells, so the cancer is not cured, but merely put on hold, but often for many years.

Intermittent hormone therapy

As the name would suggest, this involves giving an LHRH analogue for a period of time to shrink the tumour and then stopping it for a while before starting it again as the cancer starts to grow back. The thinking behind this approach is that if hormones are given constantly, the prostate cancer is going to become resistant to them quicker – a situation known as 'hormone relapse'. Furthermore, if the prostate is allowed to regenerate between the LHRH doses the prostate cancer that grows back will be more sensitive to the treatment. With this regime a LHRH analogue is used for 36 weeks and, providing the PSA has sunk below 4 ng/ml by week 32, the LHRH analogue is discontinued. The PSA is monitored as it increases until it has reached a pre-determined level when the LHRH analogue is restarted for another 36 weeks.

Survival

Studies looking at the long-term safety and effectiveness of this approach are still under way. It has been found, when studying men who have taken up to five cycles, that their prostate cancer does not seem to progress any quicker than those on continuous treatment and the patients seem to enjoy a better quality of life. More information is required however before it can be widely recommended.

Hormones followed by radical prostatectomy

Hormone therapy, in the form of LHRH implants with an initial course of anti-androgens, is used to shrink or 'down stage' the prostate cancer before carrying out a radical prostatectomy.

This approach is still being evaluated in long-term studies. Results available so far have shown that although the tumour can be shrunk, the hormone therapy does not change the Gleason score or improve survival after the operation when compared to men with similar prostate cancers who had the operation only. It has, nonetheless, shown that there is a lower incidence of positive margins (cancer at the edges of the removed prostate tissue) which signify some prostate cancer cells have been left behind after a prostatectomy. As yet this has not been adopted as a standard approach in all cases, but may be applicable in selected patients.

Hormone therapy followed by radiotherapy

Results from several large studies have shown that giving three months of hormone therapy before starting radiotherapy, usually with an LHRH analogue injection, does improve the effectiveness of treatment, with an increase in survival in men at follow-up. In the light of these positive results, many urologists and oncologists recommend this treatment strategy now. In higher risk (more advanced) cases the hormone therapy is continued for one to two years after completion of the radiotherapy.

The overall message in this chapter is that there are many different options available to men with locally advanced prostate cancer. Although the chances of cure are rather less than those men with organ-confined disease, new techniques in treatment have enabled these men to have many years free of disease and a well-maintained quality of life.

my experience

After going to my doctor with urinary symptoms I was found to have a PSA of 23 ng/ml. Biopsies revealed that I had a Gleason 4 + 4 grade prostate cancer and an MRI suggested that the tumour had invaded the capsule widely but not spread beyond. My bone scan was thankfully clear. After discussion with specialists I began hormone therapy with an injection of Prostag™ (leuprolide) and then after three months I started a seven-week course of conformal radiotherapy. I felt lucky that I only experienced modest side effects of bowel disturbance. Because I was considered to be at 'high risk' of recurrence I was advised to continue my Prostag™ injections for a further two years even though I was advised that this would effectively make me impotent. I decided that it was more important to control the cancer and decided to follow this advice.

CHAPTER

8

Treatment of metastatic disease

Unfortunately, in a proportion of men the prostate cancer escapes the gland, and secondaries develop at distant sites in the body. When a man is found to have so-called metastatic prostate cancer complete cure is not usually possible as the prostate cancer is too widespread to eliminate all of it. However, this does not mean that these men do not need specialist advice and active treatment. On the contrary, a specialist will aim to achieve prolonged control the prostate cancer to prevent further spread or deterioration in the patient's condition. Many of the methods are similar to those described in the previous chapter and we shall be referring back to these sections as the principles of hormone therapy underpin many of these interventions.

Metastatic disease refers to the situation when prostate cancer cells have broken free from the prostate gland and, having travelled in the bloodstream or lymphatics, have been deposited in other tissues such as lymph nodes or bone. In countries where PSA testing is not readily available to diagnose prostate cancer at an early

myth
Metastatic cancer is a no hope situation.

fact
This is not the case. Although the cancer is no longer curable all the specialists will try to give treatment, which increases the quantity of life for the man with prostate cancer while preserving a good quality of life.

stage, approximately one-third of men will have metastatic cancer by the time that they first consult a doctor.

Men with metastatic prostate cancer may have any of the urinary symptoms that are described in Chapter 3 as the prostate gland still has cancer in it which may cause obstruction. In addition, these men can also suffer the effects of the prostate cancer deposits in the distant non-prostate sites. The most common place by far for prostate cancer metastasis to develop is within the bones. Bone secondaries can cause pain, usually described as a constant deep-seated discomfort, in any part of the skeleton. Although any bone can be affected, the bones of the lower spine, pelvis and the ribs are most frequently affected by the deposits of prostate cancer. More unusually a prostate cancer deposit in a bone, particularly the long bones of the arm or legs, can weaken it sufficiently that a break or fracture occurs. This is known as a pathological fracture. If this happens, often as a result of only minor trauma, orthopaedic surgeons will usually be asked to advise the best way to treat the break as it can take a long time to heal. Consequently, fixation by surgery may be necessary. Other sites of prostate cancer metastasis include the liver, lung and more rarely the brain. As described in Chapter 4, if there is any suspicion of metastasis at diagnosis or at any point during treatment, scans and often tests will be performed to confirm or exclude this and the appropriate treatment started.

Treatment options and making the decision

For anyone, learning that they have prostate cancer is a huge blow. Then to find out that the cancer has spread and is no longer completely curable can induce a feeling of despair and hopelessness. The statistics can seem pretty grim; 70 per cent of men with metastatic prostate cancer will no longer be alive five years after their diagnosis. However, the positive spin on that statistic is that 30 per cent of men will be alive after five years and, furthermore, up to 10 per cent will still be alive after ten years. It is for this reason that specialists treat metastatic prostate cancer actively to give their patient as much quality time with their loved ones as they can. Moreover, there are some encouraging results of the value of chemotherapy with Taxotere™, and there are many new treatment options in the pipeline, which is improving the outlook all the time.

The treatments are largely the same as those for prostate cancer that has spread outside the gland, which were discussed in detail in the last chapter. This is because the rationale behind these treatments can also be applied to secondary prostate cancer as well. As mentioned above, metastatic deposits are small clumps of prostate cancer cells that have broken free from the prostate gland. For reasons that are not yet fully understood, these prostate cancer cells settle in another tissue, especially bone, and take root there. If you were to scrape some cells out of a metastatic deposit in some bone and look at them under the microscope they will look identical to prostate cancer cells taken directly from the prostate itself. Therefore, as they are both the same cell type they respond to treatments in the same way.

Yet again, deciding the best treatment options is an important communication exercise between the patient, any loved one or supporter that they want to involve and the team of doctors and nurses looking after their care. The treatment selected should be one that the patient is happy to accept and one that the specialist team feels is appropriate and beneficial. There is usually little point in using treatments targeted solely at the prostate gland itself as there is cancer elsewhere in the body that will be missed. The treatments are mainly based on hormone manipulation, which reduces the level of testosterone (androgen) throughout the body and stops the prostate cancer from growing and spreading no matter where it is located.

The treatment options in metastatic prostate cancer are:

✧ Bilateral orchidectomy
✧ Hormone manipulation with LHRH analogues
✧ Maximal androgen blockade using a combination of LHRH analogue and anti-androgen
✧ Maximum androgen blockade.

Bilateral orchidectomy

As described in Chapter 7, bilateral orchidectomy or surgical castration involves the removal of both testicles during a minor operation. As the testicles manufacture testosterone, a male hormone, under the control of the brain, removing them will dramatically lower the circulating levels of testosterone. As explained fully in Chapter 7, a reduced level of testosterone can stop further growth of the cancer and control it for a number of years.

The operation is usually done under a general anaesthetic where the man is unconscious, or a spinal anaesthetic where the patient feels numb from the waist down. A small cut is made in the scrotum, the blood vessels supplying the testicles are tied off and cut and the testicle is removed. There are prosthetic silicone testicles that can be put into the empty scrotum for cosmetic reasons. If the patient feels strongly that he would like this then it should be discussed prior to their admission for orchidectomy.

The main side effects of this operation are some discomfort and bruising for a couple of days after the procedure. Occasionally, a blood clot (haemotoma) can form in the scrotum, which is left to reabsorb over the next 10 to 14 days. The main advantage of bilateral orchidectomy is that it is a one-off treatment that will irreversibly lower the testosterone levels.

LHRH analogues

These are man-made chemicals very similar in composition to a substance produced in the brain called luteinizing hormone releasing hormone that stimulates the testicles to produce testosterone. At first glance it may seem illogical to give a patient something that initially increases testosterone production. However, after an initial 'flare' the testicles stop paying attention to the signals and testosterone production drops. To cover any worsening of the patient's prostate cancer during the flare a second medication is usually given temporarily. Studies have shown the level of testosterone can be reduced to a level similar to that achieved by surgical castration and that survival rates are equivalent (see Figure 8.1).

As already mentioned in Chapter 7, the LHRH analogue is given as an injection of a small pellet just under the skin or an injection into the muscles of the abdominal wall. There are one-month and three-month preparations available and usually the injections can be given through the local GP services. Although a one-month preparation is often given as a first dose, for convenience, patients are converted to the three-monthly dose as soon as possible.

The main side effects are those of hot flushes, loss of sexual drive and decreased strength of erections. The main advantage of this treatment is that the prostate cancer can be brought under control and its further growth prevented. The treatment has a fairly small impact on a man's day-to-day life with minimal hospital stays. The exact length of time the cancer remains quiescent varies from man to man and is impossible to second guess, but is usually more than one year to 18 months.

Maximal androgen blockade

Maximal androgen blockade involves treating men with advanced prostate cancers with both an LHRH analogue and an anti-androgen. Men with metastatic prostate cancer who are also relatively young and have no other significant medical problems are most likely to die because of their cancer. Studies looking at metastatic prostate cancer have shown that with LHRH analogue treatment the average time to tumour progression is 18 months with an overall survival

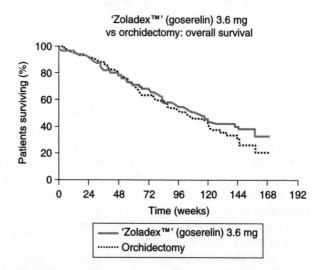

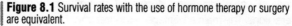

Figure 8.1 Survival rates with the use of hormone therapy or surgery are equivalent.

time of approximately 28–36 months. This is exactly equivalent to that seen with an operation to remove both testicles (see Figure 8.1). Obviously the younger, fitter men have most to lose in this situation.

Maximal androgen blockade (MAB) aims to reduce anything that stimulates prostate cancer down to a minimum. Although the overwhelming stimulus to androgen-sensitive cells is testosterone secreted by the testicles, a second chemical called androgen from the adrenal gland also plays a more minor part. It is estimated that adrenal androgen contributes 15–20 per cent and the testosterone contributes 80–85 per cent of the stimulation. The main principle behind maximal androgen blockade is that reduction of both these substances will increase the period of time to prostate cancer progression. The reason that this approach is not used in all cases is that the benefits have not been conclusively proven when compared to LHRH analogue treatment alone. Therefore the maximal androgen blockade tends to be used in the men with most to lose, that is those younger, fitter folk who would otherwise be expected to live many years.

LHRH analogues are usually the same ones given as a single agent and described extensively in the last chapter and this one. One anti-androgen that reduces the adrenal glands production of androgen is called flutamide. This is given as a daily tablet and needs to be continued for as long as it is helpful in controlling the prostate cancer.

Flutamide has one major side effect that the doctors will be aware of. In a proportion of men the liver will show signs of strain and damage as it struggles to break the flutamide down and remove it. This is monitored in the form of a blood test. If the liver shows signs of undue strain then the flutamide will be stopped to prevent

Q Why is flutamide prescribed if bicalutamide works well without any liver function disruption?

A Both these medications are just as effective on prostate cancer as each other and the risk of liver function disruption is rare. However, flutamide is more widely stocked in the UK and has certain financial advantages to the NHS. Please be assured that if there is any hint of liver damage then bicalutamide will be substituted with no questions asked.

long-term damage. An alternative, more modern anti-androgen is bicalutamide (Casodex™) which is prescribed at a dose of 50 mg per day and seldom causes liver problems.

my experience

I am 67 years old and a while ago I began experiencing urinary problems as well as back pain which was unresponsive to the usual anti-inflammatory tablets. I had my blood tested for PSA and this came back with a reading of 547 ng/ml. I had a biopsy which revealed Gleason 4 + 5 prostate cancer and a bone scan confirmed the presence of secondaries (metastases) in my skeleton. Hearing this was like a death sentence especially as I have a young wife and two small children. I went for counselling and accepted the need for hormone therapy and opted for maximal androgen blockade (MAB) with Zoladex™ (goserelin) and Casodex™ (bicalutamide) as there was some evidence that this would provide me with the best chance of survival. After therapy my PSA fell to a lowest value of 12.5 ng/ml but has recently started to rise again. I have now stopped taking Casodex™ and am currently weighing up second-line options.

Complications in metastatic prostate cancer

As metastatic prostate cancer may affect the whole body, it can cause problems in alternative areas such as the bones. Furthermore, men suffering from metastatic prostate cancer can feel weak and tired from the chronic nature of the disease. Some men lose their appetite and hence drop weight as well. If this is the case high energy and protein supplements can be prescribed, often in juice or milkshake form, to help bolster the calorie intake.

This section concentrates on two potentially serious problems that require rapid treatment. First, spinal cord compression and second, pathological fractures. Both of these are due to prostate cancer in the bone causing progressive weakness and finally collapse or breakage of the abnormally brittle bone.

Spinal cord compression

Metastatic prostate cancer has a preference for bones and especially the spinal column. When cancer deposits are concentrated in the vertebrae – the bones that sit on top of each other in a column to form the backbone – severe symptoms may develop. These bones are arranged like a stack of ring doughnuts, with the spinal cord running up the middle. The spinal cord is essentially a bundle of nerves that runs from the extremities of the body up to the brain and vice versa. If the spinal cord becomes damaged then communication between the brain and the areas of the body supplied by these nerves is interrupted (see Figure 8.2). For example, the limbs can become paralysed and feeling is lost.

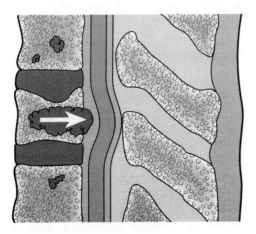

Figure 8.2 Spinal cord compression due to prostate cancer.

fact
The weakness and numbness in the legs that men experience with spinal cord compression will improve once the metastatic prostate cancer deposits are treated. The degree of improvement is dependent on how long the compression lasted. For this reason any man with prostate cancer who starts developing changes in the power and sensation in his legs should go to a hospital straightaway.

If a vertebral bone has a lot of deposits of cancer within it, it can be weakened to the point that it collapses. As it collapses the spinal cord can be squeezed because it runs through the middle, a condition called 'spinal cord compression'. Spinal cord compression causes weakness and numbness in the legs and loss of control of urinary and bowel sphincters. It is imperative that these patients attend a hospital promptly for urgent treatment as the longer the spinal cord is compressed the less likely that it will fully recover.

Treatment of spinal cord compression may be by surgery to remove the cancer that is pressing on the spine and hence relieve the pressure. If there is a nearby neurosurgical team then this will probably be the treatment undertaken. As an alternative, radiotherapy can be given, usually in combination with high-dose steroid treatment.

Following the treatment there will be a re-assessment of the hormone and other therapy the man is receiving to reduce the risk of further problems. Any other spine metastases are often treated with radiotherapy to prevent a recurrent scenario developing.

Pathological fractures

In the same way that a metastasis in the spinal bones can cause a pathological fracture, so this can happen in other bones. If the metastasis is in a long bone, such as in the arms or legs, it can snap at this weakened point. The challenge for the orthopaedic surgeons is that at the edges of this break is cancer rather than normal, healthy bone. This means that pathological fractures are less likely to heal themselves and therefore using a plaster cast to hold things in line and waiting for nature to bond the bone back together again is insufficient. Often metal work is needed to give structural support to the broken bone in the long term. This can take the form of a metal rod down the centre of the bone or a plate screwed to the outside of the bone across the fracture line. In the event that metal work is required to repair a pathological fracture, this will be inserted during an operation under an anaesthetic. Once the man has recovered from the operation, radiation is used as a back-up to slow cancer progression and prevent further problems or similar breaks in other areas. Hormone therapy is also employed if it has not been previously utilized. If it has, then second line therapy should be considered.

CHAPTER

9

When hormones no longer work

The vast majority of men with prostate cancer will receive hormone treatment at some point along their so-called 'cancer journey'. This may be the first treatment received or the hormones may be started after surgery or after radiotherapy failed to control the prostate cancer. As mentioned previously, most men on hormone therapy will eventually suffer a relapse of their prostate cancer. The most common signal of this occurrence is a progressively climbing PSA value. If the prostate cancer starts to progress despite the man receiving hormone treatment it is termed hormone relapsed prostate cancer (HRPC) (see Chapters 7 and 8).

HRPC is thought to occur as a result of hormone independent cancer cells present in the gland. As mentioned in Chapter 7, the prostate cancer cells can be divided into two main groups. The majority of the cells are hormone-dependent and will respond to normal levels of testosterone by growing and spreading. This is the fact that underpins hormone treatment; if the level of testosterone can be lowered, the hormone-dependent cells can be prevented from further growth. Unfortunately, as the normal prostate gland cells change and mutate to form cancer cells, some lose their sensitivity to testosterone. This means they will continue to reproduce and spread despite the testosterone levels being lowered by the hormone-treatment. It is these hormone-independent cells that result in hormone relapse.

Until recently men experiencing hormone relapse would be told that there was little or nothing that could be done to control the cancer. Treatments would be directed at keeping a man comfortable for whatever time he had left. Fortunately, nowadays, specialists are able to offer further treatments to try to bring the prostate cancer back under control. However, rather like hormone treatment, these further treatments are only effective for a limited period, but at least they can buy some valuable extra time for a man and his loved ones.

myth
Once the PSA starts to rise after a period of response to hormone therapy there is little more that can be usefully done.

fact
Wrong – there is now evidence that the careful use of chemotherapy agents such as Taxotere™ can result in a second remission and improve survival. Furthermore, the use of a bisphosphonate infusion at three-weekly intervals can delay the development of complications from the secondaries in the bone by an average of five months.

There are in fact several options to be considered by a man with prostate cancer. These are anti-androgen withdrawal, cytotoxic chemotherapy or bisphosphonate treatment. There is a lot of work going into the development of various new treatments such as growth factor inhibition and combination chemotherapy or gene therapy. At present these treatments are still being evaluated for their safety and effectiveness in large scientific studies. This means that they are not widely available in the UK as yet.

Anti-androgen withdrawal

When the PSA level in the blood begins to rise after a period of testosterone reduction by hormone treatment, a simple move that can be beneficial to patients is to stop some part of the hormone treatment. In some men the PSA levels will drop despite there being no active treatment. This phenomenon (which is also seen in women receiving anti-oestrogens for breast cancer) has been attributed to a mutation in prostate cancer cells. It is thought the highly abnormal prostate cancer cells have mutated so much that the anti-androgen, instead of preventing the cells from growing, in fact has the opposite, stimulating effect.

Cytotoxic chemotherapy

chemotherapy
The use of drugs to destroy cancer cells.

DNA
Short for 'deoxyribose nucleic acid', this is the substance that holds the instructions for building and repairing the body. It is found in the nucleus of each cell in our bodies.

Cytotoxic chemotherapy is what most people understand as **chemotherapy**. It is giving drugs in the form of an injection or infusion into the bloodstream or, more unusually a tablet, so killing the prostate cancer cells. Chemotherapy agents get into cells but don't destroy them instantly; instead they damage the **DNA** so that when the cell divides it dies. Chemotherapy, like radiotherapy, can't completely distinguish between normal healthy prostate cells and cancer cells. The selectiveness of the treatment relies on the fact that the cancer cells tend to divide and grow more rapidly.

The most promising agent at present is docetaxel (Taxotere™). This is an injection that is usually given at three weekly intervals.

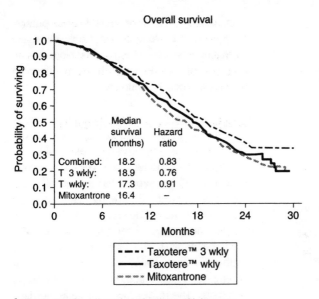

Overall survival

	Median survival (months)	Hazard ratio
Combined:	18.2	0.83
T 3 wkly:	18.9	0.76
T wkly:	17.3	0.91
Mitoxantrone	16.4	–

‐‐‐· Taxotere™ 3 wkly
Taxotere™ wkly
Mitoxantrone

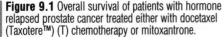

Figure 9.1 Overall survival of patients with hormone relapsed prostate cancer treated either with docetaxel (Taxotere™) (T) chemotherapy or mitoxantrone.

There have been several recent studies of the effectiveness of docetaxel that have shown that between 38 per cent and 46 per cent of men taking part had their PSA blood levels halved. Furthermore, between one-quarter and one-half of patients treated had a measurable shrinkage of the prostate cancer. Side effects include abnormalities of the blood, skin reactions and bowel upsets but overall the drug is reasonably well tolerated by the men receiving it and it can provide new hope where none was there previously (see Figure 9.1).

Oestrogens

Oestrogen (the female sex hormone) is normally found in high concentrations in the bloodstream of women. In the same way testosterone brings about the changes at puberty that make a boy a

oestrogen
The main female hormone usually found only in tiny amounts in men.

man, oestrogen is responsible for the puberty changes in girls. Normally, men only have very small amounts of oestrogen in their bloodstream. It is thought that oestrogen has two effects to prevent further prostate cancer growth and spread. First, oestrogen will stop the brain producing the hormone LHRH and thereby reduce testicular production of testosterone. The testosterone in turn can be responsible for stimulating the prostate cancer cells. The second effect is that the oestrogen has a direct effect on the prostate cancer cells, slowing their growth and resulting in some cell death.

Rather than use human oestrogen, a man-made alternative is now available called diethylstilbestrol (DES) which can be used instead. This is taken in the form of a tablet on a daily basis. The most serious side effect of DES it that it can increase the likelihood of blood clots forming in the veins of the legs (**deep vein thrombosis – DVT**) or the lungs (**pulmonary embolism**). These two conditions are the same ones that have also been linked to long haul flights. To help reduce this risk a low dose of aspirin, or less commonly warfarin, is also given daily to thin the blood and make it less likely to clot. As oestrogen is a female hormone it can cause a reduction in the growth of facial hair, and swelling in the breast area that can become tender (so-called **gynaecomastia**). Giving a dose of radiotherapy to the hormone-sensitive tissues around the nipple can often help prevent breast enlargement and nipple tenderness; this side effect is also seen with the use of anti-androgens.

Use of bisphosphonates

Bisphosphonates are a group of medicines that are used to protect the skeleton against the harmful effects of secondary cancer. They have

deep vein thrombosis (DVT)
When blood clots form in the veins of the calves. This can happen when a man is taking oestrogen tablets as they thicken the blood slightly.

pulmonary embolism
When a blood clot travels to the lungs and lodges in a blood vessel there. This can be a dangerous situation as the ability to absorb oxygen can be critically reduced.

gynaecomastia
When a man takes oestrogen the breast tissue can become tender and swell. This rarely results in noticeable enlargement and can be reduced by surgery or radiotherapy to the breast area.

been widely used in breast cancer patients for some time. Recently it has been shown that the use of a three-weekly infusion of zoledronic acid (Zometa™) can delay the development of complications of prostate cancer bone secondaries by an average of five month (see Figure 9.2). It can also reduce the symptoms of pain associated with these cancer deposits in the skeleton. Side effects are usually minor but do include a flu-like feeling at the time of the infusion.

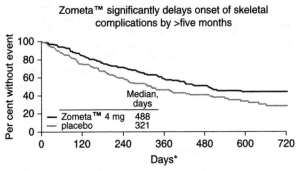

Zometa™ significantly delays onset of skeletal complications by >five months

*After start of study drug.

Figure 9.2 Bisphosphonate treatment with Zometa™ versus placebo in men with metastatic prostate cancer.

If the PSA starts to rise in a patient with prostatic cancer who has already received hormone therapy it is no longer regarded as the end of the road. There are treatments available to bring the prostate cancer back under control while still allowing a reasonable quality of life. In the event of the development of HRPC the man, his specialist team and any loved ones involved should discuss the options openly. It may be that the decision is 'no treatment' and the man should be allowed to enjoy whatever time he has left

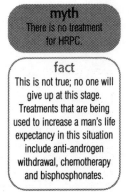

myth
There is no treatment for HRPC.

fact
This is not true; no one will give up at this stage. Treatments that are being used to increase a man's life expectancy in this situation include anti-androgen withdrawal, chemotherapy and bisphosphonates.

undisturbed. It is always important to remember that quality of life is at least as important as quantity, if not more so. The next chapter on treatment and help in the final stages of the prostate cancer journey will highlight this observation further.

my experience

I am a 61-year-old surveyor from Newcastle and began to notice that I needed to go to the toilet more often but also had difficulty passing urine. I went to my doctor and a PSA test revealed my PSA was elevated at 63 ng/ml. Biopsies confirmed prostate cancer and a bone scan confirmed secondary spread to my bones. Although I responded initially to hormone therapy with Prostap™ (leuprolide), the response only lasted 18 months and my PSA once again began to rise. I was told that there was little else to offer but I was determined not to give in and having made some enquiries and checked several websites. I requested another opinion from an oncologist with a special interest in prostate cancer. I am now receiving regular three-weekly Zometa™ (zoledronic acid) and docetaxel (Taxotere™) infusions and my PSA has shown a response, as have my symptoms of bone pain. I remain under careful review but I am not going to give up!

Local complications, such as obstruction to the ureters (the two tubular structures that connect the kidneys to the bladder), can also be resolved by the placement of plastic tubes to relieve the obstruction. If both ureters are blocked, coma from kidney failure will rapidly occur unless this is done. The decision to perform this manoeuvre should always be taken after open discussion with the patient and his family, as the question needs to be addressed as to whether it is always the right thing to do, to prolong a life which is possibly already blighted by pain and other effects of malignancy.

CHAPTER

10

Palliative care

Unfortunately, despite the best efforts on behalf of the patient by his medical team, many men's prostate cancer will eventually escape medical control and go on to cause symptoms and eventual death. **Palliative care** involves the care of the whole patient rather than solely their prostate cancer. It aims to give the man the best quality of life, free of pain and with energy, appetite and dignity. Unlike treatments from the urologist or oncologist, the palliative care team is not trying to cure the cancer, just to keep the men with cancer feeling as well as possible and positive in outlook. This often takes the form of **community based care**.

The palliative care team

This is a team of specialist doctors and nurses who have considerable expertise and experience in both the medical aspects and more practical day-to-day ones of keeping men with prostate cancer comfortable and supported. The palliative

palliative care
This becomes important in the later stages of cancer. At this point the aim of the medical teams is to make the person as comfortable as possible with the best quality of life.

community based care
This is when care and support is given to the patient either in their own home or through their local GP surgery.

care team is also there to support the family and loved ones of men with prostate cancer and to help them prepare for and face up to the loss of that person when it comes. The man with prostate cancer and his immediate family should feel that they can discuss anything that is troubling them, including spiritual or financial matters, no matter how trivial it may seem.

Each patient, as well as their family and supporters, will have the opportunity to meet the members of the team, while in hospital either as an **inpatient** or outpatient. There is a very strong team approach in this speciality with members based both in the hospital and community that are in constant communication. The most common first point of contact is in specialized cancer outpatient clinics. Within these clinics there are urologists, oncologists, radiotherapists, palliative care doctors and specialist nurses (sometimes called **Macmillan** or **Marie Curie nurses**). The aim is to make one-stop appointments where all the patient's medical and pastoral needs can be addressed.

One of the main aims of the palliative care team is to make a man with prostate cancer comfortable and positive with the best possible quality of life. They will work to keep a man out of hospital if that is what he and his loved ones want. Alternatively, they can arrange admission to a hospital or hospice to sort out specific problems or allow a period of respite. The most common problems the palliative care teams address are control of pain, treatment of bone metastases and anaemia, maintaining appetite and adequate nutrition. They also have a role in counselling patients and their family and taking measures to combat gloom, despair and depression.

inpatient
This is when the patient is admitted to a hospital ward to receive treatment and care.

Macmillan and Marie Curie nurses
Nurses who specialize in the care and support of people with cancer and their families. As a person nears the end of their life, Macmillan nurses will often be the first point of contact for any problems.

Pain and symptom control

Pain can be the most debilitating symptom of advanced prostate cancer. As well as the discomfort of the pain itself, it can be very wearing causing loss of mobility and energy, a reduction in appetite resulting in weight loss, as well as depression. A considerable amount of time and effort will be expended to optimize pain control in men with prostate cancer. There are two sides to this though, and the man with prostate cancer should tell his doctors and nurses if he is in discomfort or pain. Furthermore, if the painkiller given does not get rid of the pain the patient should not simply put up with it, but ask for something else, or a stronger dose. It can take a few attempts to get the correct type and dose of painkiller, but the palliative care team will persevere until they get it right. No man with advanced prostate cancer should be suffering unnecessary pain.

When dealing with terminal conditions, anxieties about the doses and potential addictiveness of strong painkillers is not a major issue. This is unlike when strong painkillers are prescribed to healthy people expected to survive their illness.

The progression through increasingly potent painkillers is termed the 'analgesic or pain ladder'. On the bottom rung there are painkillers suitable for mild pain which are easily available over the counter – the most commonly used is paracetamol. The next step up the ladder is paracetamol mixed with stronger painkillers such as codeine. Codeine is a weak opiate painkiller that can be very helpful in controlling moderate pain without causing too many side effects. However, codeine is not an opiate painkiller substitute, it cannot hold a candle to opiates for controlling pain. Next, pure codeine or weak

myth
Dying of prostate cancer is always painful.

fact
There will often be pain when a man with prostate cancer enters the final stages of his life. However, the medical team looking after him will not want him to suffer and will expend every effort to ensure he doesn't. Adequate painkillers will be given so that the quality of life for his remaining time will be the best it can possibly be.

opiates can be used. Nearly all the medications mentioned so far are given in the form of tablets, although suppositories and liquid preparations are available if the patient feels he is unable to swallow tablets.

At the top of the pain ladder are the **opiates**, the most common of which is morphine, although equivalents are available such as pethidine and fentanyl. Many men find the idea of taking morphine scary; they think that they will have the same high that people taking it recreationally do. They can be reassured that when opiates are taken to control pain they very rarely cause hallucinations or highs, they just relieve the pain. Some men find that they can be made a little dopey and sleepy by morphine and related painkillers – if this happens the man should let his palliative care team know, as alternative doses or preparations can be used to limit this.

One of the biggest problems with these painkillers can be constipation caused by reduction in movements of the bowel. Many doctors will give patients stool softeners or fibre preparations when they start opiates to try to prevent this. Patients should aim to open their bowels without too much of a struggle or discomfort. If there are problems, stronger laxatives or enemas can be used to get the bowels moving.

Bony metastases can cause a severe pain in badly affected bones. The most common problem areas are the lower spine and the pelvic bones, although any bone can be affected. Rather than just use painkillers to cover up the pain, one of several specific radiotherapy treatments can be used to eradicate it. These include 'hot spot' irradiation and strontium-89. Hot spot radiotherapy uses either one-off doses or a short course of radiation to the painful area.

opiates

A class of strong painkiller that is based on morphine or a man-made synthetic equivalent.

myth

Taking opiate painkillers gives you a high and turns you into a junky.

fact

It is true that if a healthy person with no pain took morphine they will get a pleasurable high and risk developing an addiction. When doctors use this strong drug to relieve pain, the body's response is different. First, as it is making pain disappear the high doesn't happen, and most patients may feel a little groggy and sleepy. Second, studies have shown that without the high and when someone is ill addiction simply doesn't happen.

In studies this treatment brought about complete pain relief in 55 per cent of men, partial pain relief in 35 per cent and only 12 per cent of men found it gave them no improvement in the pain relief.

Strontium-89 is a powerful radioactive substance that is injected into the body as a one-off in the radiotherapy outpatients department. Bone, rather than other tissues, absorbs it; furthermore bone metastases have a particular affinity to strontium, absorbing ten times more than healthy bone. Strontium lasts in the body for approximately six months and will go on being absorbed and treating bone metastases as they develop for this period. This is its main advantage over hot spot radiation that only treats a specific area. The main side effect of strontium is that it can reduce the bone marrow's normal ability to produce some of the cells in the blood. This results in a drop in the platelets – tiny structures that help blood clot. In addition, in the first two days after the injection the urine will be faintly radioactive and the patient will be given specialized containers to store urine and instructions as to how to get rid of it without risking contamination.

Home versus hospice

When a man with prostate cancer enters the final stages of his cancer journey it is often a difficult and emotional time for everyone. He will most likely be on strong painkillers and may have several other treatments to help his appetite and to keep his bowels moving. He may be too weak to move around or look after personal hygiene. The important thing to remember is that there is plenty of help available. The man's loved ones should not feel duty bound to try to do everything themselves. Help with some of the more practical

hospice

This is a place where men with prostate cancer can go to receive specialist care as he nears the end of his life. They are not hospitals. They are strong communities that can offer a lot of support to both the man and his family.

respite

This is when men with prostate cancer are admitted to a hospice for a short period of time to give their family a little break from caring for him. This is not a failure; everybody needs a chance to recharge the batteries from time to time. It can be very emotionally and physically wearing to look after a loved one with cancer.

things may give them that bit of energy and reserve to provide the emotional support to the man with advanced prostate cancer.

It is a very personal choice as to whether a patient's last remaining days or weeks are spent at home or within a **hospice**. If there is a strong desire to stay at home, then help in the form of nursing and day-to-day care is available from the Macmillan or Marie Curie charities. Hospices can also provide a short **respite** for families to give them a break from looking after their loved one. It is important at this time that the family and loved ones are there to support each other, it is not an easy time for anyone. Of course keeping people at home to die may leave a strong memory of this event inside the house. This is an area where talking to the Macmillan or Marie Curie nurse can be very important. Understandably there is going to be a wide range of emotions felt by the loved ones, some of them seemingly negative such as anger and resentment. This is natural and nothing to feel ashamed about. It is best discussed and brought out into the open.

The alternative is that the man with prostate cancer is admitted to a hospice. This is not in any way an abandonment or easy route out. To some, the supportive environment of the hospice with other people and their families in a similar situation can be comforting and supportive. Many hospices are also well supported by local communities of various faiths which some find eases the emotional burden. Often the palliative care team will discuss hospice care with the man with prostate cancer and his family a little before it is needed. This gives them a chance to go and visit the local hospice and discuss and decide if this is a service they wish to take up. Nobody will mind if the patient or their family changes their

myth
Knowing someone will die makes it easier.

fact
We wish this was the case but in fact knowing death will happen does not make it easier. Families of men with prostate cancer will feel a huge range of emotions from anger to relief and grief. Some can feel guilty that selfish emotions such as 'why me?' or relief are felt but they won't be the first or last person to go through this. Losing a loved one is a difficult experience that no one can prepare for. The grieving process is personal and each person has to work through their emotions until they reach a point of acceptance. Finding support in family and friends to talk things through can help hugely. Alternatively, counsellors, Macmillan or Marie Curie nurses can give support at this difficult time.

mind at any time – last-minute admissions or discharges can be arranged as needed.

Losing a loved one is never easy and, despite what is sometimes stated, knowing that someone will inevitably die does not make it easier when that day comes. The palliative care team is there to support the patient and his family through the final stages of the illness. All the support will be aimed at keeping the patient comfortable and ensuring both his and his family's last wishes are followed as far as is possible. They will also be able to support the family just after the death of the man to help guide them down the road of acceptance and eventual recovery.

CHAPTER

11

Taking control

Everyone is an individual and each person's experience of prostate cancer is different. We hope that having read this book you will see that tackling prostate cancer requires a team effort with several different types of doctors, specialist nursing staff and other support workers, working together as a team to provide the best treatment. The crucial members of this team are the man with prostate cancer and those family members that he wishes to involve in his care. Decisions are joint ones, with the patient having a crucial say in which of the options he would like to pursue. As we have often mentioned, not all the options will apply to every man and not every treatment will be available in every unit but everything can be discussed.

It is undeniable that a diagnosis of prostate cancer can be difficult to deal with. Some people react by denial, others with anger and resentment. These are all natural emotions and will often pass with time. Eventually people find their way to acceptance. Nobody wants to face up to his or her own mortality, but the key to coping is to make the most of the time left. These reactions are not just limited to the man receiving the diagnosis of prostate cancer, their family and other loved ones will also go through the same emotions.

It is widely accepted that it is better to talk openly about a diagnosis of cancer and share hopes and fears with people. Some men feel that they should be strong and protect their loved ones by not telling them about their prostate cancer. 'What they don't know won't hurt them' is something all doctors have heard their patients say. However, most of the time the family have guessed that something is wrong and can be hurt that they have been excluded during such a stressful event. Furthermore, once treatment has started it is difficult to hide the time spent in the hospital for surgery or radiotherapy or the need to take regular medication. Although it is only one person who has the prostate cancer, the whole family and circle of friends will be affected by it and it is better that they deal with whatever happens together and with open communication.

At the end of the day it is up to the man with prostate cancer himself to decide upon the best course of action for him. A doctor or nurse should not talk to any relative or friend about the diagnosis, treatment or prognosis of any medical condition without the express permission of the patient concerned. Therefore, if there are specific facts that a man wishes to remain private and personal he should point this out to his doctor and the team. The doctor may enquire why, and maybe point out some of the pitfalls or problems with withholding information, but will always respect the final decision of the patient. Of course this works both ways and a doctor, nurse or counsellor will answer any questions a patient has fully, truthfully and to the best of their knowledge. Relatives and friends may think it is kinder to withhold certain unpleasant facts from the patient, but a doctor may not tell lies at their request.

Finally, there is a vast amount of information about prostate cancer. Books, websites and articles in the press are all easily available (see page 133). However, there is a wide variability in the accuracy and scientific basis of the information available and if you have any doubts discuss them with your doctor and his team. As a general rule, information presented through a recognized charity or scientific institution is the most reliable and tends to be written in plain English with non-medically qualified people in mind. There is also a lot of information about prostate cancer research, particularly on the web, which should be treated with some caution. The problem is that the treatments and breakthroughs lauded on these sites are often still experimental and relatively untested and it may be many years before these are translated into proven, commercially available treatments.

Time management and appointments

It is a good idea for the man with prostate cancer to bring along a family member or close friend to his hospital appointments. This is more than the practical help of someone to arrange transport and to chat to while hanging around waiting for the allotted appointment time. The appointments will often involve discussion with a large number of facts being given to the patient. It is very difficult for one person to absorb all the information so quickly and therefore two or more sets of ears are often better than one.

Another good tip is to take along a pen and paper to jot things down as the appointment proceeds. If the same pad is used each time it will become a reference guide to how that patient's treatment has developed and progressed and can be referred to during appointments. Questions that the patient and family may think of between appointments can also be noted down here so that when they get to see the specialist they remember to ask them.

A diary is another useful tool. Very quickly a number of appointments to see various specialities and to attend for tests and scans can build up. Although the hospital will send out letters to confirm these dates, keeping a diary with it all in one place is a little easier to deal with. It also means that the well-organized patient can sometimes arrange to have a scan and other test appointments on the same day to cut down travelling and time wasted.

It should be remembered that the treatment of prostate cancer, such as radiotherapy may be tiring and patients can find it increasingly energy-sapping to attend the hospital. This is where the companion really comes into their own, to escort patients to the hospital, find out where they need to go and wait for them. Most hospitals do have wheelchairs for the use of patients while in the hospital so they can cut down on the amount of walking, although finding one can sometimes be a challenge!

Overall, prostate cancer will often have a major effect on the man's life and all those who love him. Remember though that there are lots of people out there to help. The medical team and nurses will do everything they can to cure the prostate cancer. For those men who unfortunately have incurable prostate cancer the focus will be on keeping the cancer under control for as long as possible and allowing the man to carry on living his life to the full. The charities and organizations listed in 'Further help', (page 133) all offer support, information and practical advice. Many of the people involved in these charities have either had a diagnosis of prostate cancer themselves or have supported someone else through their treatment. No matter how unique and isolated someone may feel, invariably there will have been someone in the same situation that can empathize. Just remember no one needs to fight prostate cancer by themselves – you are not alone – just ask for help and it will usually be forthcoming.

CHAPTER

12

Sex and the prostate

As has already been mentioned, prostate cancer in almost all its stages and various manifestations can potentially have a very adverse effect on the sex life of the patient. Moreover, almost all the treatment options employed to manage the disease will have an impact on this very important facet of a man's life and secondarily upon that of his partner.

So what are the most common conditions affecting a man's sex life and his prostate?

Sexual dysfunction in men can have a range of causes involving not only physical, but also psychological factors. In fact, it is difficult to separate the two since successful sexual interaction involves both the mind and the body working together. Some of the most common male sexual problems experienced by men with prostate cancer are:

✧ **Erectile dysfunction** ('ED' or 'impotence') – the medical term for difficulty in achieving or keeping a satisfactory erection for a fulfilling sex life.

✧ **Ejaculation problems** – including premature (early) ejaculation, delayed ejaculation and retrograde ejaculation. Retrograde ejaculation is when a man experiences an orgasm, but there doesn't seem to be any fluid as it has gone back into the bladder rather than come out of the penis. The fluid will come out the next time he urinates.

✧ **Reduced sexual desire (libido)** – resulting from various psychological or physical problems depending on age, sex, sexual history and other factors.

libido
The medical term for the sex drive or desire to have sex. A lot of the treatments for prostate cancer will reduce the libido.

Table 2 Prostate cancer treatments linked to sexual problems.

Treatment	Potential sexual side effects
Hormone treatments	Erection problems and decreased libido
Surgery	Retrograde ejaculation and erection problems
Radiotherapy	Erection problems

TURP
This is short for transurethral resection of prostate. This is an operation during which the middle of an enlarged prostate gland is removed piecemeal by an instrument inserted up through the penis to help a man pass urine.

Transurethral resection of the prostate (**TURP**) is commonly performed for the treatment of BPH (benign prostatic hyperplasia – see Chapter 5) but much less commonly performed for prostate cancer. The portion of the prostate that is blocking the urethra (the tube that carries urine from the bladder) is removed by hot wire resection via an instrument inserted down the urethra.

The sexual side effects associated with a TURP can include semen that flows backward into the bladder during ejaculation (retrograde ejaculation) as well as erection problems, although erection problems aren't always directly associated with the surgery. Recently Greenlight™ and Holmium™ laser prostate resection is becoming more popular. Laser technology means that prostate tissue can be removed in an almost bloodless way, and the catheter can be removed after 24 hours, or sooner. Because laser energy does not penetrate beyond the capsule, erectile dysfunction is uncommon but retrograde ejaculation still often occurs.

Many of the sexual side effects that result from prostate cancer or the treatment initiated for it can be treated effectively. One of the problems is that very often men and their partners receive only sparse information about the problems they might encounter or the potential solutions for them.

While libido is difficult to improve without boosting testosterone (androgen) levels, which would carry a risk of reactivating the androgen-dependent cancer, erectile dysfunction will often respond to a number of treatment strategies. These include:

✧ Phosphodiesterase type 5 inhibitors (PDE5I) which improve the rigidity of erections by slowing the breakdown of nitric oxide (NO) within the penis. Available drugs include Viagra™ (sildenafil), Cialis™ (tadalafil) and Levitra™ (vardenafil).
✧ Intraurethral prostaglandin E1 in the form of medicated urethral system for erection (MUSE).
✧ Intracorporeal prostaglandin E1 (Caverject Dual Chamber™) which is the most effective approach, but is associated with some discomfort and a risk of bruising and a prolonged response which discourages many patients.
✧ Surgical implantation of silicone prostheses into the penis. These devices, which come in semi-rigid and inflatable varieties provide an erection sufficient for intercourse. They may be applicable in men with early stage disease, however they are seldom used in patients with more advanced tumours who have frequently lost their sex drive.

myth
Loss of erections cannot be helped.

fact
There are several treatments to help restore a man's erections that are safe to take in conjunction with treatment for prostate cancer. Furthermore, as the erection problems are the result of the prostate cancer and its treatment, these therapies can be obtained on an NHS prescription.

As in many other aspects of the prostate cancer journey a holistic approach is required. With a proactive approach many of the sexual difficulties encountered by prostate cancer patients can be improved. A sympathetic and understanding approach is required from all the health care professionals involved in the management including specialists, nurse practitioners and GPs. This understanding should be extended not only to the patient but to his partner whose quality of life may also be seriously affected by the disease or the effects of its treatment. From the patient or his partner's point of view, the key thing is not to be ashamed or embarrassed to raise the question. Effective treatment is now available for many sexual problems, so don't be afraid to ask.

my experience

I have prostate cancer which was treated several years ago with a radical prostatectomy. Although the surgeon told me that he had saved the nerves, after the operation I could not get an erection. At first I was embarrassed to discuss this either with my wife or the medical team, but eventually I plucked up the courage. I am so glad I did because the prostaglandin injections really worked and now I can function well simply with a tablet of Viagra™. As a result I feel that I have not lost my manhood.

CHAPTER

13 Future developments in diagnosis and treatment

With the increasing awareness of the sometimes devastating effects of prostate cancer it has begun to attract ever greater academic attention and considerably more research funding. Those people working with and for men with prostate cancer, who had felt it was a Cinderella subject as far as basic research is concerned, have enthusiastically received this and genuine progress is now being made.

Chemoprevention

Much work is being done to try to find substances that will prevent the development of prostate cancer. There is some evidence that vitamin E and selenium supplements may reduce the likelihood of prostate cancer. There is no definitive evidence that these supplements are effective but many men choose to take them as they have few side effects.

There is another major trial underway that is giving men a medication called dutasteride

(Avodart™). These men will be monitored for many years to see if the group taking dutasteride has a lower rate of prostate cancer when compared to men not taking it. Unfortunately, the answer will not be available for several years.

Earlier detection

Obviously detecting a prostate cancer earlier will mean a higher proportion of men could have curative treatment. The advent of PSA testing (see Chapter 5 for more details) has already improved the situation. As Chapter 5 points out PSA is not exclusive to prostate cancer and unfortunately non-cancerous problems in the prostate gland can also increase the PSA level. Much work has been done to improve the accuracy of this test in diagnosing prostate cancer. One of the ways is using free to total PSA ratios or the new UPM3 urine-based test. A great deal of work has examined alternative markers of prostate cancer and certain genes that may point to prostate cancer developing, and the future of these technologies looks bright.

Prognostic indicators

As we target resources to diagnosing cancer at an earlier stage when it is a potentially curable organ confined prostate cancer, we are finding very small tumours. The treatments for organ defined prostate are removal or destruction of the prostate gland and these do have significant side effects. Therefore it would be sensible to try to find a way to identify those cancers that are going to grow rapidly and aggressively so treatments can be targeted specifically to those men. There are several molecules in prostate cancer samples that are showing promise as ways to identify the more aggressive cancers. These include E-Cadherin, anti-cathepsin B and protein EZH2. Others are in the pipeline and look promising.

New therapies

At present radical prostatectomy and radiotherapy are the main stays of treatment for organ-confined prostate cancer. However, both of these treatments have significant side effects affecting erections and continence of urine. There are new techniques to try to minimize the risks of these by using **laparoscopic** (keyhole surgery) techniques, **cryotherapy** to freeze the gland and the use of **high intensity focused ultrasound (HIFU)** energy. Robotic assistance for laparoscopic radical prostatectomy is also being evaluated and may well improve outcomes.

Other novel strategies are looking at controlling the prostate cancer that has spread outside of the prostate gland. As well as refining the existing hormone manipulation treatment, the LHRH analogues new treatments are also being developed. Promising candidates at the moment include growth factor inhibitors and chemicals that prevent prostate cancers forming new blood vessels to bring in nutrients. Two further compounds exisulind (Aptosyn™) trastuzumab (Herceptin™) are already being tested in men with prostate cancer although there is no answer yet as to whether they are safe and effective or not.

Gene therapy

The recent spectacular advances in molecular biology have made the prospect of safe and effective gene therapies an imminent reality. Gene

laproscopic
A technique where surgery is done via a series of small cuts in the abdomen, which allow the passage of a camera and instruments. The main advantage of laproscopy (sometimes called keyhole surgery) is it is less invasive than conventional techniques and patients recover quicker. Prostatectomy can now be performed laproscopically by urologists trained in the technique.

cryotherapy
The prostate gland is frozen to destroy the cancer cells it contains. The probes are inserted through the perineum during an operation.

high intensity focused ultrasound (HIFU)
This uses the energy from ultrasound to destroy the prostate gland and the cancer it contains.

therapy for prostate cancer is most likely going to proceed down one of the following avenues:

✧ Getting control of the cell's excessive division rate causing its growth
✧ Introducing cancer-killing substances into cancer cells while leaving adjacent healthy prostate cells unaffected
✧ Developing vaccines to stimulate the body's own immune system to attack and destroy prostate cancer cells.

The prospects for significant advances in the struggle against prostate cancer in the near future are good. As well as research into preventing prostate cancer in the first place, work continues to allow earlier and more accurate diagnosis and there are also continuing improvements in the effectiveness of treatments and the reduction in the side effects. Whatever the future holds, the battle to reduce the death rate and complication rate of prostate cancer seems set to intensify. We hope that this book will empower the reader and his or her family to join the fight to defeat this most prevalent and debilitating disease which touches so many peoples' lives.

Further help

Cancer BACUP
3 Bath Place
Rivington Street
London
EC2A 3JR
Information service: 020 7613 2121
Free helpline: 0808 800 1234
www.bacup.org.uk

Cancerlink
11–21 Northdown Street
London
N1 9BN
Free helpline: 0808 808 0000

The Continence Foundation
307 Hatton Square
16 Baldwins Gardens
London
EC1N 7RJ
Helpline: 020 7831 9831 (09.30–16.30
Monday to Friday)
www.continence-foundation.org.uk

Cancer Research UK
P.O. Box 123
Lincoln's Inn Fields
London
WC2A 3PX
Tel: 020 7121 6699
www.cancerresearchuk.org

The Impotence Association
PO Box 1029
London
SW17 9WH
Helpline: 020 8767 7791
www.impotence.org.uk

Macmillan
Macmillan Cancerline
Macmillan Cancer Relief
89 Albert Embankment
London
SE1 7UQ
Tel: 0208 808 2020
www.macmillan.org.uk

Marie Curie Cancer Care
89 Albert Embankment
London
SE1 7TP
Tel: 0207 599 7777
www.mariecurie.org.uk

The Men's Health Forum
Tavistock House
Tavistock Square
London
WC1H 9HR
www.menshealthforum.org.uk

NHS Direct
Tel: 0845 4647
www.nhdirect.nhs.uk

Patient UK
www.patient.co.uk

The Prostate Cancer Charity
3 Angel Walk
London
W6 9HX
Helpline: 0845 300 8383
www.prostate-cancer.org.uk

Prostate Research Campaign UK
10 Northfields Prospect
Putney Bridge Road
London
SW18 1PE
Helpline: 0207 877 5840
www.prostate-research.org.uk

Glossary

active surveillance This is when a man is monitored closely and his symptoms controlled but no treatment is given to the prostate cancer. It is aimed at keeping quality of life high and is frequently used in older men or those with medical conditions that would limit their life expectancy.

age related cut-offs These are a set of slowly increasing upper limits of 'normal' PSA range with advancing age.

anaemia The medical term for having a low blood haemoglobin level. Anaemia can cause tiredness and shortness of breath on exertion.

anaesthetist A doctor that specializes in putting patients to sleep prior to surgery and waking them up after, and who is also in the control of pain.

anastomosis The medical term for the joining back together of two cut ends of tube when a length has been removed at surgery. An anastomosis is performed in the urethra during a radical prostatectomy.

androgens These are the hormones, or chemical messengers, that are particularly linked to the male sexual

characteristics and organs. The most well known
of the androgens is testosterone.

anti-androgens Drugs which block the action of testosterone on
the body and hence are also used in hormone
therapy.

benign prostatic A benign or non-cancerous condition that
hyperplasia (BPH) causes the prostate gland to swell up. BPH, like
prostate cancer, can cause difficulty in passing
urine.

benign tumour A growth that, although increasing in size outside
of the body's control, can't invade the
surrounding structures or spread elsewhere
inside the body.

biopsy The removal of a small sample of any body
tissue for analysis. Biopsies are usually taken to
see if there is cancer present or not.

bone scan Radioactive markers are used to show up whether
there are prostate cancer deposits in the bone
and, if so, where they are.

brachytherapy A type of radiotherapy that uses radioactive
pellets implanted directly into the prostate gland.

catheter A narrow tube inserted into the penis and up to
the bladder to drain urine away. The tube is
connected to a bag that will collect the urine as it
drains. Catheters can be used temporarily after
operations or in the longer term if required.

cavernous nerves These are the nerves that initiate erections in
men. The nerves run alongside the prostate
gland and can be damaged during a radical
prostatectomy.

chemotherapy The use of drugs to destroy cancer cells.

chromosome Each cell has 23 paired rod-like chromosomes
which are responsible for the transmission of
hereditary characteristics.

community based This is when care and support is given to the
care patient either in their own home or through their
local GP surgery.

cryotherapy The prostate gland is frozen to destroy the cancer
cells it contains. The probes are inserted through
the perineum during an operation.

CT (computerized tomography) scan	A method of using sequential X-rays to build up a three-dimensional picture of the body.
deep vein thrombosis (DVT)	When blood clots form in the veins of the calves. This can happen when a man is taking oestrogen tablets as they thicken the blood slightly.
differentiation	When healthy prostate is seen under the microscope a pathologist will easily recognize it as coming from the prostate gland. This is 'well differentiated' tissue. As cancer takes over, the prostate cancer cells can lose some of their characteristic prostate features. These cells are now 'poorly differentiated' and unrecognizable from any other cancer.
digital rectal examination (DRE)	This allows the doctor to assess the size and texture of a man's prostate gland. It involves placing a gloved and lubricated finger in the man's back passage to feel the gland.
DNA	Short for 'deoxyribose nucleic acid', this is the substance that holds the instructions for building and repairing the body. It is found in the nucleus of each cell in our bodies.
ejaculation	The emission of about a teaspoonful of sperm with a nourishing fluid at the point of orgasm.
ejaculation problems	These include premature (early) ejaculation, delayed ejaculation and retrograde ejaculation. Retrograde ejaculation is when a man experiences an orgasm but there doesn't seem to be any fluid as it has gone back into the bladder rather than come out of the penis. The fluid will come out the next time he urinates.
epidural	A technique an anaesthetist may use to control pain during and after an operation. An injection of local anaesthetic is put around the spinal cord to numb the body from that level down.
erectile dysfunction ('ED' or impotence)	This is the medical term for difficulty in achieving or keeping a satisfactory erection for a fulfilling sex life.
external genitalia	The medical term for the sexual organ, comprising the penis, scrotum and testicles in a man.
first degree relative	This is basically your parents or your brothers and

sisters, providing they have the same parents. In the case of prostate cancer, a disease seen in men only, we are only interested in fathers and brothers.

flare phenomenon
When a man is first started on an LHRH analogue there is an initial surge in testosterone levels before they drop. To protect against stimulation of the prostate cancer during this period a short course of anti-androgens is given.

free to total PSA ratios
A method that attempts to make PSA more predictive of prostate cancer. PSA can be bound to a protein in the blood but when there is prostate cancer the amount of unbound PSA in the bloodstream increases. Therefore the ratio will increase.

frequency
The need to empty the bladder at regular intervals during the day. The amount of urine may be large or small.

genes
These are the smaller building blocks of chromosomes. There are millions in every chromosome. Each gene can be responsible for forming a specific characteristic, chemical or protein within the body.

Gleason grading system
Developed by Dr Gleason, this is an international system of grading how abnormal prostate cancer cells look under the microscope. The grades run from 1 to 5, and the higher the grade the more aggressive a cancer it is likely to be.

Gleason score
Prostate cancer is not uniform in Gleason grade. Therefore it is common to note the grades of two areas in the biopsy sample, for example, $2 + 2 = 4$. Again, the higher the score the more aggressive the prostate cancer is likely to be.

grading
This looks at the prostate cancer cells themselves to assess how aggressive the prostate cancer is likely to be.

gynaecomastia
When a man takes oestrogen the breast tissue can become tender and swell. This rarely results in noticeable enlargement and can be reduced by surgery or radiotherapy to the breast area.

haemospermia This is where blood is mixed in with the sperm and is seen once it has been ejaculated at the time of orgasm. It can be a sign of prostate cancer but also of stones or an infection in the urinary system.

hesitancy The term for the situation when a man has to wait seconds or minutes at the toilet to start urinating, despite him feeling he wants to go. Often men strain to pass urine at this point.

high intensity focused ultrasound (HIFU) This uses the energy from focussed ultrasound to destroy the prostate gland and the cancer it contains.

hormone relapsed prostate cancer (HRPC) A prostate cancer that has started to grow and spread again after a period of control on hormone therapy.

hormone therapy The use of drugs to block the stimulatory effects of testosterone on the growth of the prostate tissue and hence slow down the spread of prostate cancer.

hormones Chemical messengers that travel through the bloodstream. Hormones allow different bits of the body to communicate with each other. Usually hormones influence processes at a different site from where they are produced.

hospice A place where a man with prostate cancer can go to receive specialist care as he nears the end of his life. They are not hospitals. They are strong communities that can offer a lot of support to both the man and his family.

impotence This is when there is a problem in gaining any erection or one strong enough for penetrative intercourse.

incomplete emptying The feeling that urine remains in the bladder despite the fact the man has stopped passing urine.

incontinence The uncontrolled leakage of urine at any time other than when you urinate. It can be a small amount due to a weakness in the sphincter or complete loss of control if the sphincter is badly damaged.

inpatient
This is when the patient is admitted to a hospital ward to receive treatment and care.

intermittency/post micturition dribbling
When the stream of urine stops and starts and finishes with dribbles and drips rather than cleanly.

intermittent hormone therapy
This is cycling between periods of hormone treatment and periods of rest from the treatment to try to increase a man's quality of life while still controlling the prostate cancer.

IPSS
The International Prostate Symptom Score is a standardized questionnaire that specialists may ask a man to fill out so they may assess how bad the urine symptoms are.

jaundice
The yellow discoloration of the skin that occurs when the liver cannot do its job of clearing toxins from the body. Metastases from prostate cancer can cause a failure of the liver as they replace the normal tissue.

laparoscopic
A technique where surgery is done via a series of small cuts in the abdomen, which allow the passage of a camera and instruments. The main advantage of laparoscopy (sometimes called keyhole surgery) is it is less invasive than conventional techniques and the patient recovers quicker. Prostatectomy can now be performed laproscopically by urologists trained in the technique.

LHRH analogues
Luteinizing hormone releasing hormone analogues are drugs that switch off the production of testosterone by the testicles. They are used in hormone therapy.

libido
The medical term for the sex drive or desire to have sex. A lot of the treatments for prostate cancer will reduce the libido.

linear accelerator
This is a machine that allows the focused delivery of radiation to the prostate gland. It looks a bit like an X-ray machine and the patient lies on a table in the middle of the machine to receive his treatment.

local spread	When the prostate cancer grows and breaches the capsule of the prostate gland and spreads into the surrounding tissues.
locally advanced disease	Prostate cancer that has spread outside the surrounding capsule of the prostate gland but has not, as yet, spread to distant areas in the body through the bloodstream.
luteinizing hormone	This is produced by the brain and travels in the bloodstream to the testicles where it tells them to start producing testosterone.
lymph nodes	These occur at regular intervals throughout the lymphatic system and act as small filters, so cells such as cancer cells tend to accumulate at these points. The swollen glands you get in your neck during the flu are an example of lymph nodes.
lymphatic system	This system of small vessels drains fluid (lymph) from the body's organs, filters it and returns it back to the bloodstream.
Macmillan and Marie Curie nurses	Nurses who specialize in the care and support of people with cancer and their families. As a person nears the end of their life, Macmillan nurses will often be the first point of contact for any problems.
malignant tumour	The medical term for what is commonly called cancer. In malignant tumours the uncontrolled cancer cells are invading normal surrounding healthy tissue and have the potential of forming metastases. A malignant tumour has the ability to kill a person.
maximal androgen blockade	This is using LHRH analogues and anti-androgen at the same time to prevent a prostate cancer progress.
metastases	This is when cancer cells travel through the bloodstream or the lymphatic system to other parts of the body and settle there. The word secondaries is often used instead of metastases.
modifiable risk factors	Risk factors that a man can do something about, for example, stopping smoking, losing weight or eating a healthy diet.

MRI scan	This stands for magnetic resonance imaging. This builds a three-dimensional reconstruction of the body. Unlike a CT scan, MRI detects very small movements in the bodies cells when they are exposed to a magnet for a short period of time.
nanograms per millilitre (ng/ml)	This is a measure of concentration that is used in PSA tests. The PSA figure is in fact the amount of PSA in nanograms seen in 1 millilitre of blood.
nocturia	The need to get up and pass urine multiple times during the night despite cutting down on the amount drunk of an evening.
non-modifiable risk factors	Risk factors that a man can't change despite his best intentions. For example, his age, family history or race.
oestrogen	The main female hormone usually found only in tiny amounts in men.
oncologist	A doctor that specializes in the medical treatment of cancer.
opiates	A class of strong painkiller that is based on morphine or a man-made synthetic equivalent.
orchidectomy	The surgical removal of both testicles to reduce the amount of testosterone in the body. Orchidectomy is an irreversible form of hormone therapy.
organ-confined disease	A prostate cancer that is buried within the prostate gland with no spread outside of it. This means that if the prostate gland is removed during surgery or destroyed by radiation the cancer can be cured.
outpatients	This is when you travel to a hospital to consult with a specialist at a booked time. It does not require you to stay in hospital.
palliative care	This becomes important in the later stages of cancer. At this point the aim of the medical teams is to make the person as comfortable as possible with the best quality of life.
pathological fractures	A break through an area of bone weakened by a prostate cancer metastasis.
pathologist	A doctor who specializes in looking at the structure of tissues microscopically. Pathologists

play an important role in diagnosing and guiding the treatment of cancer.

perineum
The area of skin situated behind the scrotum and in front of the anus.

PIN
Prostatic intraepithelial neoplasia can only be diagnosed by a pathologist looking at a sample of prostate tissue. In PIN, the prostate cells look abnormal but crucially have not started to invade surrounding healthy cells and hence become cancer. Although not technically a cancer, PIN is often seen as a forerunner to cancer.

prostate gland
This is a chestnut sized (20 cc) organ found only in men. It sits just below the bladder and surrounds the urethra or tube that drains the bladder through the penis. Its job is to produce a substance that liquefies the jelly-like substance that sperm are stored in so they can swim towards and fertilize the egg.

protective factors
Things that may protect a man from getting prostate cancer, for example taking selenium and vitamin E supplements.

PSA (prostate specific antigen)
PSA is a protein produced by all prostate glands whether healthy or not. If the prostate has a cancer in it or is inflamed because of infection, the amount of PSA detected in the blood rises. To help diagnose prostate cancer and monitor its response to treatment, doctors use PSA readings in the form of a blood test.

PSA density
The PSA reading divided by the volume of the prostate gland. It is a method to try to make PSA tests more predictive for prostate cancer.

PSA velocity
The rate of year on year increase of the PSA level. It is thought an increase of more than 0.75 a year is likely to be due to prostate cancer.

pulmonary embolism
When a blood clot travels to the lungs and lodges in a blood vessel there. This can be a dangerous situation as the ability to absorb oxygen can be critically reduced.

radical prostatectomy
An operation for prostate cancer in which the prostate gland, seminal vesicles and some of the

nearby lymph nodes are removed. It is an option in fit men when the cancer is confined to the prostate gland.

radiotherapy
The use of radiation to kill cancer cells. With external beam radiotherapy the radiation is generated from an external source and focused on to the prostate.

referral
A process where one doctor asks a fellow doctor, usually of a different speciality, to review a patient and offer help in their diagnosis or treatment.

respite
This is when a man with prostate cancer is admitted to a hospice for a short period of time to give his family a little break from caring for him. This is not a failure; everybody needs a chance to recharge the batteries from time to time. It can be very emotionally and physically wearing to look after a loved one with cancer.

risk factor
Anything that increases the chances of a man getting prostate cancer compared to a similar man in absence of the risk factor.

second degree relative
This is anyone once removed from the first degree relatives, for example grandparents, aunts and uncles. In prostate cancer we are interested in the male second degree relatives.

seminal vesicles
A pair of storage vessels for sperm, found just behind the prostate gland and often one of the first areas that prostate cancer spreads to.

signs
These are the changes in the body, caused by a disease, which a doctor will pick up as he or she examines the patient. Some are easy to see or feel as they are on the surface of the body, for example, a swelling in the groin. Some involve an internal organ that may need special scans or tests to pick up.

spinal cord compression
This is when a bony metastasis in the spine compresses the cord containing the major nerves that run through it. It will result in loss of sensation and power in the legs and sometimes loss of bladder and bowel control.

staging	This looks at how far a prostate cancer may have spread outside the prostate gland.
symptoms	These are the problems that men with prostate cancer notice that prompt them to go to see a doctor. Symptoms are often regarded as a change from the normal. With prostate problems, the commonest symptom people suffer from is increasing difficulty in passing urine and the need to visit the toilet more often, especially at night. Discomfort develops as a result of incomplete bladder emptying.
testosterone	The hormone responsible for many male characteristics. It has a role in stimulating growth of prostate tissue, so some drugs used in prostate cancer work by disrupting its production or effect.
transrectal ultrasound scan (TRUS)	An ultrasound method that allows the prostate to be seen. It involves inserting a lubricated probe into the back passage to visualize the prostate gland. It is used to guide biopsies or brachytherapy treatment.
tumour	A collection of cells that increases in number outside the body's normal control. Tumours may be cancerous or non-cancerous (benign).
TURP	This is short for transurethral resection of prostate. This is an operation during which the middle of an enlarged prostate gland is removed piecemeal by an instrument inserted up through the penis. It is done to help a man pass urine.
urgency	A sudden overwhelming desire to empty the bladder. People often think they are on the verge of wetting themselves and will run to the toilet. Other men describe urgency as suddenly feeling like they have more urine in their bladder than they could possibly hold.
urologist	A doctor that specializes in disorders affecting the kidneys, bladder and, in men, the prostate.
weak stream	A reduction of the force and strength of the stream as a man passes urine. It tends to be a gradual decline in the force over time.

Sources of figures and plates

Figure 1.1
The anatomical location of the prostate gland.

Figure 1.2
The anatomy of the prostate gland.

Figure 1.3
Areas of the body to which prostate cancer can metastasize (spread) –
the lymph nodes, lungs and bones.

Figure 4.1
Digital rectal examination of the prostate.

Figure 4.2
Transrectal biopsy of the prostate.

Figure 4.3
Transrectal ultrasound scan showing a prostate tumour.

Figure 4.4
Clinical staging of prostate cancer.

Figure 6.1
PSA recurrence after radical prostatectomy: supersensitive assays will
reveal recurrence earlier.

Figure 6.2
Radical prostatectomy versus watchful waiting. Holmberg et al, 2002.

Figure 6.3
Conformal radiotherapy more accurately targets the prostate.

Figure 6.4
Brachytherapy involves implantation of radioactive seeds into the prostate.

Figure 6.5
Cryotherapy aims to destroy cancer cells by freezing with cryotherapy needles.

Figure 6.6
First, second and third generation cryotherapy needles. The third generation probes produce a more even ice ball to destroy cancer within the prostate.

Figure 7.1
The action of drugs which are used in prostate cancer.

Figure 8.1
Survival rates with the use of hormone therapy or surgery are equivalent. Kaisary et al, 1991.

Figure 8.2
Spinal cord compression due to prostate cancer.

Figure 9.1
Overall survival of patients treated with hormone relapsed prostate cancer treated either with docetaxel (Taxotere™) (T) chemotherapy or mitoxantrone. Petrylak et al, 2004.

Figure 9.2
Bisphosphonate treatment with Zometa™ versus placebo in men with metastatic prostate cancer. Saad et al, 2002.

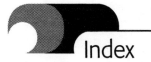

Index

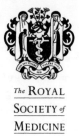

The ROYAL
SOCIETY of
MEDICINE

The Royal Society of Medicine (RSM) is an independent medical charity with a primary aim to provide continuing professional development for qualified medical and health-related professionals. The public benefits from health care professionals who have received high quality and relevant education from the RSM.

The Society celebrated its bicentenary in 2005. Each year it arranges and holds over 400 meetings for health care professionals across a wide range of medical subjects. In order to aid education and training further the Society also has the largest postgraduate medical library in Europe – based in central London together with online access to specialist databases. RSM Press, the Society's publishing arm, publishes books and journals principally aimed at the medical profession.

A number of conferences and events are held each year for the public as well as members of the Society. These include the successful 'Medicine and me' series, designed to bring together patients, their carers and the medical profession. In addition the RSM's Open and History of Medicine Sections arrange meetings on a regular basis which can be attended by the public.

In addition to the lectures and training provided by the RSM, members of the Society also have access to club facilities including accommodation and a restaurant. The conference and meeting facilities of the RSM were refurbished for their bicentenary and are available to the public for hire for meetings and seminars. In addition, Chandos House, a beautifully restored Georgian townhouse, designed by Robert Adam, is also now available to hire for training, receptions and weddings (as it has a civil wedding licence).

To find out more about the Royal Society of Medicine and the work it undertakes please visit www.rsm.ac.uk or call 020 7290 2991. For more information about RSM Press, please visit www.rsmpress.co.uk.